DECISION MAKING SERIES

PSYCHIATRIC DECISION MAKING

STEVEN L. DUBOVSKY, M.D.

Associate Professor of Psychiatry and Medicine
Associate Dean for Academic Affairs
University of Colorado School of Medicine
Denver, Colorado

ALAN D. FEIGER, M.D.

Department of Psychiatry
Lutheran Hospital
Wheat Ridge, Colorado

BEN EISEMAN, M.D.

Professor of Surgery
University of Colorado School of Medicine
Chairman, Department of Surgery
Rose Medical Center
Denver, Colorado

Distributed by
YEAR BOOK MEDICAL PUBLISHERS • INC.
35 EAST WACKER DRIVE, CHICAGO

1984

B. C. DECKER INC. • Philadelphia • Toronto
The C. V. MOSBY COMPANY • Saint Louis • Toronto • London

Publisher: **B.C. Decker Inc.**
3228 South Service Road
Burlington, Ontario L7N 3H8

B.C. Decker Inc.
Six Penn Center Plaza, Suite 305
Philadelphia, Pennsylvania 19103

North American and worldwide sales and distribution:

The C.V. Mosby Company
11830 Westline Industrial Drive
Saint Louis, Missouri 63141

In Canada: **The C.V. Mosby Company, Ltd.**
120 Melford Drive
Toronto, Ontario M1B 2X5

Psychiatric Decision Making

ISBN 0-941158-16-0

Library of Congress catalog card number: 83-72418

Last digit is print number: 10 9 8 7 6 5 4 3 2 1

With grateful appreciation and thanks to
William Bernstein, M.D., Lynn Feiger, and Joshua Feiger

CONTRIBUTORS

NEIL J. BAKER, M.D.

Assistant Professor, Department of Psychiatry, University of Colorado School of Medicine, Denver, Colorado

DEBORAH COYLE, M.D.

Instructor, Department of Psychiatry, University of Colorado School of Medicine, Denver, Colorado

STEPHEN DILTS, M.D., Ph.D.

Associate Professor, Department of Psychiatry, University of Colorado School of Medicine; Chief of Inpatient Services, Denver General Hospital, Denver, Colorado

STEVEN L. DUBOVSKY, M.D.

Associate Professor of Psychiatry and Medicine, Associate Dean for Academic and Faculty Affairs, University of Colorado School of Medicine, Denver, Colorado

ALAN J. FEIGER, M.D.

Clinical Instructor, Department of Psychiatry, University of Colorado School of Medicine, Denver, Colorado

RONALD D. FRANKS, M.D.

Associate Professor, Department of Psychiatry, University of Colorado School of Medicine, Denver, Colorado

CARL J. GETTO, M.D.

Assistant Professor of Psychiatry, Associate Dean for Clinical Affairs, University of Wisconsin School of Medicine, Madison, Wisconsin

WILLIAM V. GOOD, M.D.

Assistant Professor, Department of Psychiatry, University of Colorado School of Medicine, Denver, Colorado

ERIC HADDES, Ph.D.

Director, Sleep Laboratory, Presbyterian Hospital, Denver, Colorado

DANIEL A. HOFFMAN, M.D.

Clinical Instructor, Department of Psychiatry, University of Colorado School of Medicine, Denver, Colorado

ROBERT M. HOUSE, M.D.

Assistant Professor, Department of Psychiatry, University of Colorado School of Medicine, Denver, Colorado

JOYCE S. KOBAYASHI, M.D.

Assistant Professor of Psychiatry, University of Colorado School of Medicine; Director of Liaison Psychiatry, Denver General Hospital, Denver, Colorado

MARJORIE W. LEIDIG, Ph.D.

Clinical Psychologist; Adjunct Faculty, Department of Psychology, University of Colorado, Boulder, Colorado; Former Clinical Director, Battered Women Research Center, Denver, Colorado

JEFFREY L. METZNER, M.D.

Assistant Clinical Professor of Psychiatry, University of Colorado School of Medicine, Denver, Colorado

MICHAEL G. MORAN, M.D.

Assistant Professor, Department of Psychiatry, University of Colorado School of Medicine, Denver, Colorado

PETER PARKS, M.D.

Lutheran Hospital Emergency Service, Wheatridge, Colorado

JANICE L. PETERSEN, M.D.

Assistant Professor, Department of Psychiatry, University of Colorado School of Medicine, Denver, Colorado

EUGENE SCHWARTZ, Ph.D.

Boulder, Colorado

GREGORY STEINWAND, Psy.D.

Boulder, Colorado

TROY L. THOMPSON, II, M.D.

Associate Professor of Psychiatry and Medicine, University of Colorado School of Medicine, Denver, Colorado

WENDY L. THOMPSON, M.D.

Assistant Clinical Professor, Department of Psychiatry, University of Colorado School of Medicine; Department of Medicine, National Jewish Hospital, Denver, Colorado

PREFACE

Recent developments in psychiatry, like those in other medical specialties, have had a profound effect on the ways in which scientific information is acquired. Expanded knowledge now accumulates so rapidly that even the subspecialist has difficulty finding the time to review all of the new developments in his field. Generalists in psychiatry, and practitioners in other fields who must keep themselves informed about a number of specialties, increasingly are finding that remaining informed about the broad scope of psychiatric knowledge is a formidable task indeed. This book was written for the busy practitioner who needs a rapid review and an opportunity to update his or her conceptualizations.

As is true of any clinical field, an approach to a psychiatric problem has two components. The first consists of actual facts, techniques, and interventions, many of which change with breathtaking speed. The second and more enduring component concerns the conceptual framework that defines the overall approach to a disorder. Clarification of this approach is of great assistance in developing a tangible structure that is open to discussion, development, and growth. As computerized instructional formats have facilitated more exact simulations of the clinical setting, educators have realized that the ways in which clinical problems are analyzed and solved need more emphasis than they have received. *Psychiatric Decision Making* is meant to be a forerunner of a new generation of works that study the form as much as the content of clinical thinking.

No matter how subjective some psychiatric problems may seem, it is usually possible to objectify the process by which clinical decisions are made. The algorithms in this volume summarize approaches to most common psychiatric problems of adults and children. These highly succinct summaries are meant to encourage the experienced clinician to objectify and review his or her own approach in a way that will facilitate incorporation of new information as well as straightforward discussions with colleagues and students. The clinician who is less familiar with the treatment of a particular disorder should, in a few minutes, be able to understand how at least one authority approaches that problem. We have included approaches of varying complexity in an attempt to make this book useful to practitioners with differing levels of expertise and interest in psychiatry.

Since our intention was to formalize the overall approach to complex clinical phenomena rather than to review the finer points of management and theory, we had to sacrifice a certain amount of detail in order to provide a format that allows the reader to integrate a number of ideas at a glance. Once these basic treatment assumptions are clarified, further reading of more detailed texts and the literature should expand the clinician's understanding readily. As in any field, disagreements with the approaches advocated by this particular group of authors are inevitable and healthy; but seeing one method objectified should at least help the reader to make it plain exactly in what ways and why he or she would do things differently.

The authors of the algorithms in this book initially were skeptical about condensing a great deal of information and experience into a small space. However, they eventually decided that brevity may be more likely to be an indication of expertise than of ignorance. We hope that well versed readers will enjoy reviewing and formalizing their own approaches and that newcomers will develop a basic framework that will facilitate further learning.

This book could not have been written without the dedicated and expert technical assistance of Peg Robbins and Maxine Peterson. We are also extremely grateful to Mary K. Maudsley and Brian Decker for their encouragement, help, and forbearance.

We acknowledge the support and encouragement of Philip and Ilse Feiger and the challenge to creativity and productivity constantly provided by Doug Carter.

Steven L. Dubovsky, M.D.
Alan D. Feiger, M.D.
Ben Eiseman, M.D.

CONTENTS

PSYCHIATRIC ASPECTS OF MEDICAL CARE

SLEEP DISORDERS

ORGANIC BRAIN SYNDROMES

SUBSTANCE ABUSE

SEXUAL DYSFUNCTIONS

How To Use This Book

Depending on its complexity, each clinical topic is discussed in one or more algorithms. Essential baseline data are described before the point at which the first decision must be made. The algorithm branches at crucial decision points. Notes on the page facing the algorithm elucidate points that require further discussion or debate. The approach presented reflects each author's clinical experience and his or her understanding of the literature; the references are meant to provide further background reading. A few chapters in the form of tables summarize diagnostic criteria and the use of various psychotropic medications. The latter information is, of course, highly subject to modification, and the reader should reconfirm preparations and dosages from additional sources before prescribing them.

Each algorithm is meant to address the decision making *process* more than the *content.* As such, it is a skeleton upon which the flesh of more detailed clinical and theoretical knowledge can grow. The greatest benefit will therefore be obtained when the reader focuses on his or her own broad approach to a clinical problem, comparing and contrasting it with that of the chapter's author. Since each decision tree focuses more on the structure of a clinical decision than on its content, additional reading is necessary to develop a well rounded understanding of each clinical problem.

THE ANGRY PATIENT

Ronald D. Franks, M.D.

COMMENTS

A. Patients may express anger overtly, or as noncompliance, continued complaints, or nonpayment. If anger is understood as an attempt to communicate a problem, it is easier to avoid responding with anger of one's own. Anger that is uncharacteristic of the patient is likely to be due to an acute interpersonal or intrapsychic disturbance.

B. Acknowledgement that the patient has a right to be angry with lapses on the part of the physician, his staff, and ancillary personnel often reduces the patient's need to complain angrily in his attempt to make the physician understand his distress. If anger persists despite correction of realistic complaints, the patient is likely focusing on the physician anger derived from another situation.

C. Anger originally directed toward a spouse, boss, or previous physician may be displaced (transferred) onto the physician. This transference may result in the expectation that the doctor, like some other person in the patient's experience, will be rejecting, controlling, or angry or will fail to meet the patient's needs. Anger may also be a means of avoiding anxiety or other emotions aroused by illness. Sometimes the patient is angry with the physician for not curing him, or with himself for being ill. Pointing out that the patient's past experiences may make it seem that the current physician will treat him as other people have, may help the patient to recognize the difference between present and past situations. Open discussion of the patient's feelings about his illness and its treatment, and of current interpersonal conflicts, helps him to understand his feelings and gain more control over them, reducing helplessness, fear and anger.

D. Acute anger that does not respond to discussion of current stresses and transference may be caused by more serious psychiatric disorders, especially depression (pp 56–57), mania (pp 42–43), acute psychoses (pp 30–31), or schizophrenia (pp 36–37), which require more extensive evaluation and treatment.

E. Chronically angry behavior often reflects a lifelong (characterologic) way of interacting that may decrease but is not likely to be relinquished entirely.

F. If the patient becomes angry when he is dependent on or close to others as a means of increasing interpersonal distance, the patient's opinion about all aspects of treatment should be solicited and excessive displays of friendliness (e.g., calling the patient by his first name) should be avoided.

G. The patient with an underlying sense of inadequacy may attempt to bolster self-esteem by treating the physician with angry disdain. Conveying the attitude that the patient is an important person diminishes fears of being ridiculed by a powerful and important person.

H. Patients whose chronic anger worsens when the doctor is not readily available are usually afraid of rejection and loneliness and use anger to hold onto the physician. Being readily available to the patient (e.g., answering calls promptly and seeing the patient regularly) may allay these fears.

I. Continued anger may reflect the patient's perception that the doctor does not like him. Since it is virtually impossible to work effectively with a patient who does not evoke any positive reactions, the patient who arouses only dislike should be helped to find another physician. If no other physician is available, consultation with a colleague is necessary to help the doctor minimize the effects of his own feelings on his medical decisions.

J. It is important to prevent the patient's behavior from alienating or exhausting the doctor. The patient should be told that he may discuss his feelings in words but cannot express them in

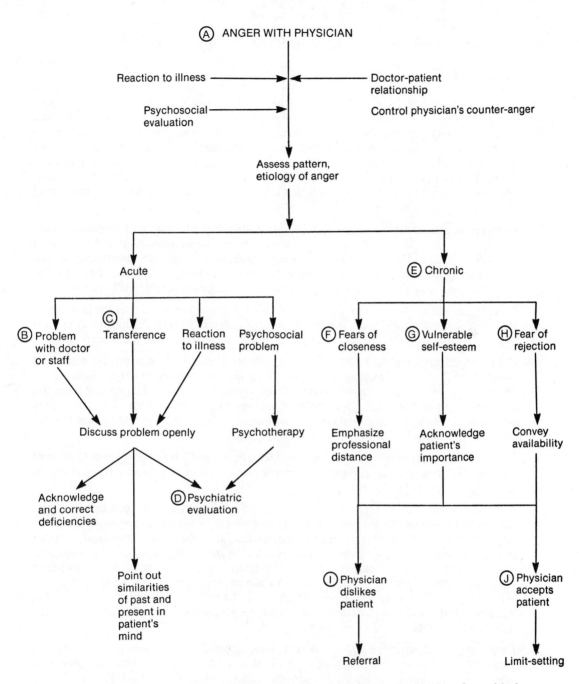

A ANGER WITH PHYSICIAN

Reaction to illness ───────→ ←─────── Doctor-patient relationship

Psychosocial ──────────→ Control physician's counter-anger
evaluation

Assess pattern,
etiology of anger

Acute   **E** Chronic

B Problem   **C** Transference   Reaction   Psychosocial   **F** Fears of   **G** Vulnerable   **H** Fear of
with doctor   to illness   problem   closeness   self-esteem   rejection
or staff

Discuss problem openly   Psychotherapy

Emphasize   Acknowledge   Convey
professional   patient's   availability
distance   importance

Acknowledge   **D** Psychiatric
and correct   evaluation
deficiencies

Point out   **I** Physician   **J** Physician
similarities   dislikes   accepts
of past and   patient   patient
present in
patient's
mind

Referral   Limit-setting

destructive ways. If the patient cannot control behavior that threatens to interfere with the physician's neutrality, treatment should be terminated.

REFERENCES

Franks RD. Working with angry patients. Amer Family Physician 1981; 24(5):123–125.

Groves JE. Taking care of the hateful patient. N Engl J Med 1978; 298:883.

Kahana RJ, Bibring GL. Personality types in medical management. In: Finberg NE, ed. Psychiatry and Medical Practice in a General Hospital. New York: International University Press, 1964: 108.

Lipsitt DR. Medical and psychological characteristics of "crocks". Psychiatry Med 1970; 1:15.

DENIAL OF ILLNESS

Troy L. Thompson II, M.D., and Robert House, M.D.

COMMENTS

A. Denial is a defense mechanism that reduces anxiety by keeping out of conscious awareness the seriousness of an illness or even its existence. Denial early in the course of an illness is a common means of giving oneself time to adjust to a frightening reality, especially if the condition is unexpected, life-threatening or has important symbolic meaning. Apparent unawareness of the implications of an illness may also represent an attempt to reassure the family. Diseases of the nondominant hemisphere may be associated with denial of associated neurologic disturbances. Any condition that impairs memory may produce apparent denial due to forgetting.

B. If the patient is somewhat aware of a condition that frightens him and protection from anxiety is only partial, attempts to reduce anxiety further through increased denial may lead the patient to avoid treatment entirely. Such a mechanism may be responsible for the reluctance to seek prompt medical attention after experiencing symptoms of myocardial infarction, and may lead to the high incidence of sudden death outside the hospital.

C. Reassurance that he will receive good care without stressing the dangers of the illness may help the patient to seek appropriate treatment. Persistent anxiety leading to continued avoidance of therapy may be reduced by short-term administration of antianxiety drugs.

D. If the patient states that he is not seriously ill but cooperates with treatment, denial of the extent of the illness should not be challenged. Treatment alternatives should be discussed in a way that does not arouse excessive anxiety about side effects or other dangers and is not too insistent on his demonstrating a complete understanding of his problem. The family may need to be helped to understand the protective nature of the patient's denial and not to force complete acknowledgment of the situation too quickly.

E. If the patient is not competent to refuse treatment, he generally is not competent to consent and a guardian should be appointed to protect his rights once a court has ruled on the question of competence (pp 10–11).

F. If the danger is likely to pass in a reasonably short time, it may be possible to secure temporary compliance by asking the patient to consent to treatment for a specified period to satisfy the physician or the family and not because the patient believes he is seriously ill. If the patient continues to refuse necessary care because he does not believe that he is sick, his defenses may need to be temporarily overwhelmed in order to secure at least short-term cooperation while antianxiety medications are administered to control the resulting panic sufficiently for the patient to continue treatment. If the patient's life is in imminent danger, lifesaving treatment may be administered against the patient's will (pp 10–11); legal consultation should be obtained.

G. Denial in medical patients is seldom due to a major mental disorder. These patients therefore are usually legally competent and cannot be forced to comply with nonemergency care even if noncompliance eventually will lead to serious disability or death (pp 10–11).

H. Denial of the seriousness of an illness may lead to failure to carry out important tasks (e.g., making a will) in addition to refusal to cooperate with treatment. If the task can be separated from the illness (e.g., by emphasizing that everyone needs a will), the patient may view it as an ordinary event rather than an indication of the severity of his illness. Confrontation when immediate compliance is not urgently needed is likely to increase denial; the physician should remain available but allow the patient to decide when he wishes to seek information or treatment.

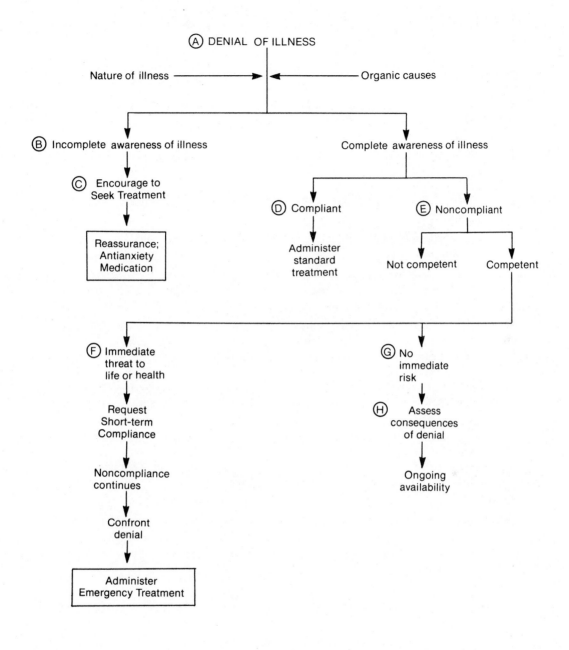

REFERENCES

Weisman AD. Coping with illness. In: Hackett TP, Cassem NH, eds. Massachusetts General Hospital Handbook of General Hospital Psychiatry. St. Louis: CV Mosby, 1978: 264–275.

Dubovsky SL, Weisberg MP. Clinical Psychiatry in Primary Care. 2nd ed. Baltimore: Williams & Wilkins, 1982.

Strain JJ, Grossman S. Psychological Care of the Medically Ill. New York: Appleton-Century-Crofts, 1968: 23–36.

Hamburg DA. Coping behavior in life-threatening illness. Psychother Psychosom 1974; 23:13–25.

Blumenfield M, Thompson TL. Psychological reactions to physical illness. In: Simons RC, Pardes H, eds. Understanding Human Behavior in Health and Disease. 2nd ed. Baltimore: Williams & Wilkins, 1981: 46–56.

FAILURE TO PAY FOR SERVICES

Ronald D. Franks, M.D.

COMMENTS

A. The delinquent patient may have forgotten or be unwilling to pay, or may be attempting to call the physician's attention to a previously unrecognized problem, often in the doctor-patient relationship.

B. Patients who find it difficult to keep up their accounts may be identified by a past history of difficulty with bills, behavioral disturbances, or angry, unsatisfactory relationships with physicians. Explaining the physician's charges and billing practices in advance and asking if the patient anticipates any difficulties with financial arrangements may help to avoid later problems.

C. Angry reactions or minimization of problems may make it difficult to identify and confront issues that lead to a failure to pay.

D. Personal contact to ask whether nonpayment reflects a problem the patient has not discussed serves as a reminder that the treatment contract is with the physician, not with an impersonal office or system the patient does not feel obligated to pay.

E. Patients experiencing financial problems may feel so overwhelmed even by moderate bills that they make no attempt to pay. Reassuring them that a manageable monthly payment is acceptable often helps them to regain self-esteem and continue regular contact with the physician. If this does not provide sufficient relief, a decreased frequency and/or duration of appointments may reduce costs to an acceptable level. Exploring reluctance to apply for financial assistance is indicated when problems are severe.

F. Failure of patients with borderline (pp 140–141), antisocial (pp 138–139) or other personality disorders to keep their accounts current may reflect a wish to be cared for without taking responsibility for themselves or a wish to test the physician's ability to limit their behavior. Failure to insist on payment may result in fear that the physician cannot control them and increased actions that are destructive of the physician's good will may result.

G. When nonpayment reflects dissatisfaction with therapy or other causes of anger with the physician, guidelines for management of the angry patient (pp 2–3) are applicable.

H. Failure to pay may be a covert means of encouraging the physician's curiosity in the hope that undiscussed symptoms will be uncovered.

I. The wish not to pay until he feels better may represent an attempt to control anxiety and helplessness through the illusion that recovery can be guaranteed by controlling payment. Empathy, allowing the patient some control over his treatment, education about his illness, and ongoing physician availability may be sufficiently reassuring.

J. Crises in the patient's life may be alleviated by seeing the patient regularly for 4 to 6 weeks to help him express emotions, define conflicts, and find new adaptive solutions.

K. Occasionally, nonpayment alerts the physician to a serious underlying psychiatric disorder that may be revealed by questioning the patient about unusual experiences, thoughts, feelings and about use of drugs. If vigorous treatment does not result in an improved sense of responsibility, the patient may be communicating a wish to be declared disabled and unable to meet his obligations.

L. If the patient has noted frightening new symptoms, nonpayment may be a means of avoiding the physician while calling attention to himself through his behavior.

M. Unless arrangements for reduced fees or free care are the result of careful discussion with the

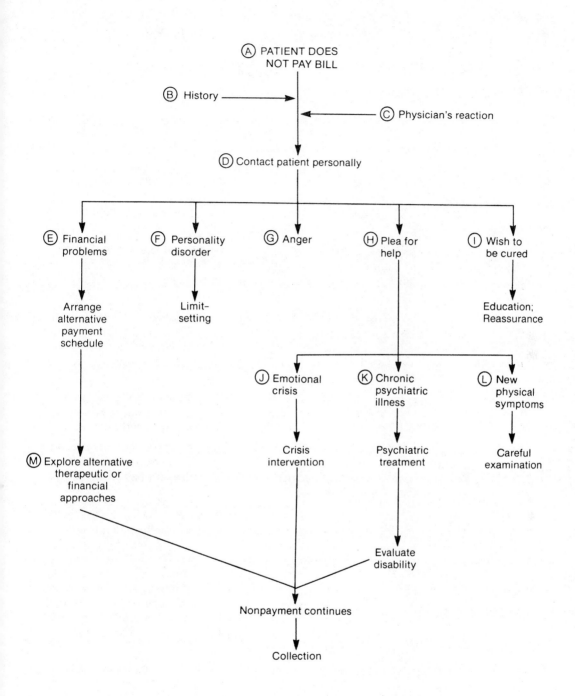

patient, allowing continued nonpayment is likely to arouse anger, loss of self-esteem, and concern about why the doctor does not value the treatment. Although the physician may terminate treatment for a nonemergency condition, he should help the patient to find alternative care.

REFERENCE

Bird B. Talking with Patients. Philadelphia: JB Lippincott, 1955.

NONCOMPLIANCE

Troy L. Thompson II, M.D.

COMMENTS

A. Noncompliance should be expected when a patient has a history of noncompliance, expresses signficant doubts about the recommended treatment, does not respond to treatment that should be effective, or reveals fears of medications.

B. Therapeutic instructions, the risks of noncompliance and the benefits of treatment should be reviewed in concrete language and repeated by the patient, to confirm that he understands why the treatment has been recommended and that he is capable of following instructions. The patient's feelings about the therapeutic regimen and the doctor should be discussed routinely, if only briefly.

C. The regimen should be as simple as possible, organized around daily rituals (meals, bedtime), given in the least possible number of doses by a family member or friend. There may be a need to prescribe less expensive alternatives and to investigate possible sources of financial support.

D. Impairment of hearing, vision, or memory, lack of education, low intelligence, cultural and language barriers may result in failure to comprehend instructions fully; denial (pp 4–5) may lead to noncompliance. Patients may benefit from written instructions, medication logs and pill packs in which the day and time for each pill is clearly noted. Denial may be reduced by reassurance and avoidance of confrontation.

E. If transient unpleasant side effects occur, either the patient can be encouraged to continue taking the medications until these diminish, or the dose can be reduced. If side effects persist or are particularly disturbing, changing to a different medication may be indicated.

F. Noncompliance reflecting anger at the physician or his staff (pp 2–3) may be caused by real or imagined lapses in efficiency or compassion, disappointment, or may be an attempt to resist the physician's influence or to control him. Open discussion may help the patient express his concerns in words instead of noncompliance.

G. Depression may cause noncompliance if the patient is pessimistic about the chances of improvement or if he is covertly attempting suicide. The patient should be reminded that hopelessness is a symptom of depression which should be treated vigorously. The hypochondriacal patient may unconsciously wish to remain ill; reassurance that he will continue to be considered sick may help. Extreme hopelessness, delusions of poisoning, suspiciousness, and reluctance to give up the euphoria of mania may lead to outright noncompliance or to the more subtle "cheeking" of medications in psychotic patients. Close supervision of therapy, which may be against the patient's will (pp 10–11) is often necessary. Malingerers and patients with factitious disorders avoid therapy because they do not want their simulation uncovered; empathic confrontation may help to solve their problems.

H. When the patient's ability to comply is impaired, involvement of the family is crucial to encourage the patient, assist with the regimen, monitor compliance and uncover reasons for noncompliance.

REFERENCES

Blackwell B. Drug therapy: patient compliance. N Engl J Med 1973; 289:249–252.
Diamond RS. Enhancing medication use in schizophrenia. J Clin Psychiatry 1983; 44:7–14.
Francis V, Korsch B, Morris MJ. Gaps in doctor-patient communication. N Engl J Med 1969; 280:535–540.
Gillum RF, Barsky AJ. Diagnosis and management of patient noncompliance. 1974; JAMA 228:1563–1567.
Haynes RB. A critical review of the "determinants" of patient compliance with therapeutic regimens. In Sackett DL, Haynes RB (eds). Compliance with Therapeutic Regimens. Baltimore, Johns Hopkins Press, 1976, pp 26–39.

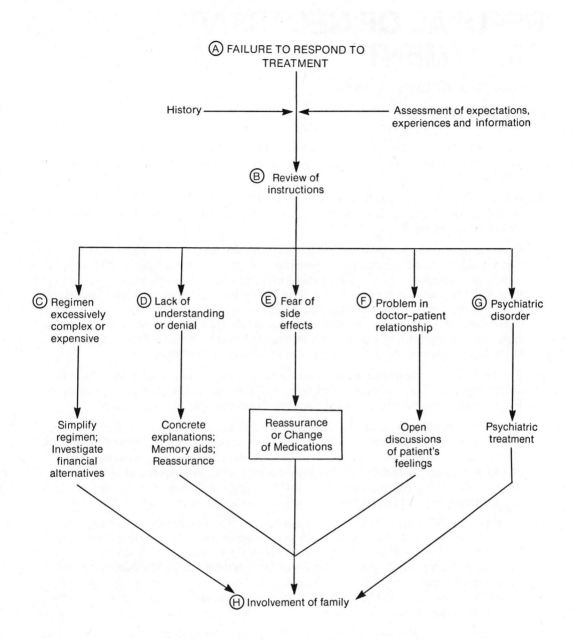

Ⓐ FAILURE TO RESPOND TO
TREATMENT

History ⟶ ⟵ Assessment of expectations,
experiences and information

Ⓑ Review of
instructions

Ⓒ Regimen
excessively
complex or
expensive

Ⓓ Lack of
understanding
or denial

Ⓔ Fear of
side
effects

Ⓕ Problem in
doctor-patient
relationship

Ⓖ Psychiatric
disorder

Simplify
regimen;
Investigate
financial
alternatives

Concrete
explanations;
Memory aids;
Reassurance

Reassurance
or Change
of Medications

Open
discussions
of patient's
feelings

Psychiatric
treatment

Ⓗ Involvement of family

Stoudemire A, Thompson TL II. Medication noncompliance: systematic approaches to evaluation and
    intervention. Genl Hosp Psych 1983; 5:233–239.
Becker MH, Maiman LA. Strategies for Enhancing Patient Compliance. J Comm Health 1980; 6:113–135.
Haynes RB. A critical review of the "determinants" of patient compliance with therapeutic regimens. In:
    Sackett DL, Haynes RB, eds. Compliance with Therapeutic Regimens. Baltimore: Johns Hopkins
    Press, 1976: 26–39.
Matthews D, Hingson R. Improving patient compliance—a guide for physicians. Med Clin North Am 1977;
    61:879–889.
Hulka BS, Cassel JC, Kupper LL, et al. Communication, compliance and concordance between physicians
    and patients with prescribed medications. Am J Pub Health 1976; 66:847–353.

REFUSAL OF NECESSARY TREATMENT

Joyce S. Kobayashi, M.D.

COMMENTS

A. Active refusal of indicated treatment is relatively rare; passive refusal of long-term therapy by noncompliance may occur up to 50% of the time, especially among lower socioeconomic groups.

B. A physician may treat an immediately life-threatening medical emergency or order diagnostic procedures that might confirm the presence of a life-threatening injury or illness, even if the patient refuses consent.

C. If the patient refuses treatment in which the potential benefit is relatively low compared to the risk, consideration of the patient's objections is warranted. If the relative danger to the patient of refusing therapy is great, he is more likely to be declared incompetent by a court than if the benefit of treatment is less certain. Psychotic patients or those involuntarily committed to psychiatric wards may still be competent to refuse treatment. Once the court determines incompetence, a guardian (often a family member or close friend) must be appointed to consent to the patient's treatment and protect his interests. Ongoing discussions of the patient's reasons for refusal often lead to his eventual consent.

D. Patients may refuse treatment because of concerns about pain, loss of function, or because of uncertainty regarding an unproven new therapy. Family members, friends, or even fictional TV characters may have reported adverse experiences that frightened the patient.

E. Refusal of treatment may also reflect the patient's feelings about the doctor. For example, if the patient feels that the physician does not like him or does not inform him sufficiently, he may lack sufficient confidence to agree to treatment. Refusal may also express anger (pp 2–3) or a wish to assert control of the physician. Encouraging open expression of the patient's concerns, correcting realistic complaints, and pointing out feelings that are inappropriate may help the patient to feel sufficiently confident in the physician.

F. Depressed patients may feel that nothing can help them and there is no point in agreeing to treatment; if they are covertly suicidal, they may refuse treatment because they want to die. A few psychotic patients have delusional ideas about the treatment or the doctor. Vigorous treatment of the underlying disorder usually overcomes their refusal. Malingerers who refuse treatment that could expose their dissimulation should be confronted (pp 8–9). Hypochondriacal patients should be reassured that they will not lose contact with the physician if they improve (pp 84–85).

G. Consultation with the patient's family and others may reveal cultural beliefs that favor folk remedies, or family objections to the recommended course. Asking the patient to describe his understanding of the treatment may uncover a language difficulty that interferes with the patient's understanding. The patient may also feel unable to afford treatment.

H. Noncompliance may be prevented by continued inquiry about the patient's feelings about therapy. A competent patient should not be coerced into compliance; however, the physician may refuse to treat a noncompliant patient. The patient's immediate safety should be ensured and reasonable attempts made to find another doctor.

REFERENCES

Stone AA. Mental Health and Law: A System in Transition. Rockville, Maryland: NIMH, 1975.
Janicak PG, Bonavich PR. The borderland of autonomy: medical-legal criteria for capacity to consent. J Psychiatry Law 1980; Winter: 361–386.

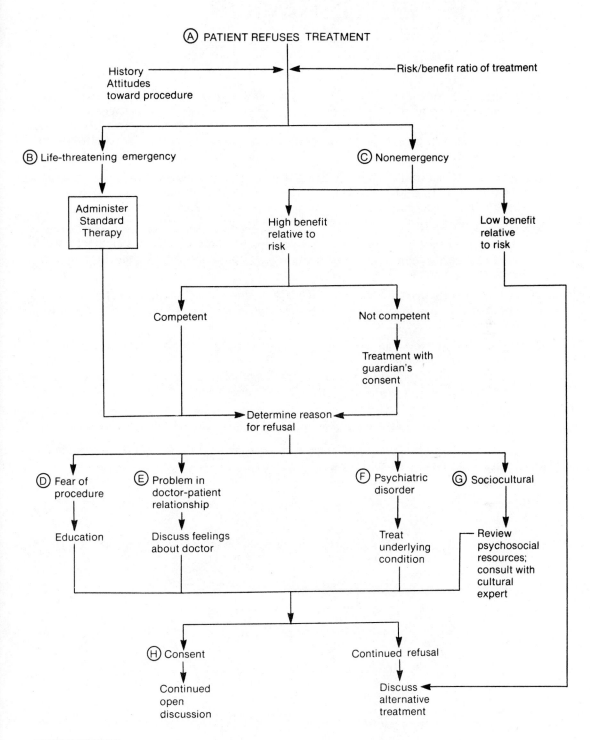

A PATIENT REFUSES TREATMENT

History ——————————→ ←—————————— Risk/benefit ratio of treatment
Attitudes
toward procedure

B Life-threatening emergency   C Nonemergency

Administer   High benefit   Low benefit
Standard   relative to   relative
Therapy   risk   to risk

                    Competent   Not competent

                                                 Treatment with
                                                 guardian's
                                                 consent

                              Determine reason
                              for refusal

D Fear of   E Problem in   F Psychiatric   G Sociocultural
procedure   doctor-patient   disorder
                 relationship

Education   Discuss feelings   Treat   Review
                 about doctor   underlying   psychosocial
                                            condition   resources;
                                                               consult with
                                                               cultural
                                                               expert

              H Consent   Continued refusal

              Continued   Discuss
              open   alternative
              discussion   treatment

REFERENCES

Roth LA, Lidz C. Tests of competency to treatment. Amer J Psychiatry 1977; 134:279–284.
Beeker MH. Understanding patient compliance: the contributions of attitudes and other psychosocial factors. In: Cohen SJ, ed. New Directions in Patient Compliance. Lexington, Massachusetts: DC Heath & Co, 1979: 1–31.

SEDUCTIVE BEHAVIOR

Ronald D. Franks, M.D.

COMMENTS

A. Regardless of how obvious it may be to the physician, most seductive behavior is not apparent to the patient. Rather than a request for a sexual encounter, seductiveness that is out of keeping with the patient's usual behavior is an attempt to communicate distress about an acute problem, especially an interpersonal crisis, sexual dysfunction, illness affecting the patient's attractiveness or sexuality, loss of self-esteem, or depression.

B. For heterosexual seductiveness, finding better solutions to recent stresses usually decreases the need to signal distress through seductiveness. There is no need to discuss sexuality at length with the patient unless the underlying problem is a sexual dysfunction.

C. Patients who habitually behave in a seductive manner usually do not benefit from extensive discussions of their behavior; rather, they may feel encouraged to become more seductive if the doctor pays attention to their seductiveness. The physician should ignore their advances and proceed with the medical workup.

D. If seductive behavior continues, the patient should be told emphatically but firmly that the physician can be of more service professionally than sexually and that sexual advances are unacceptable in the doctor's office.

E. If the physician is not homosexual, homosexual seductiveness is likely to arouse anxiety and anger. As with heterosexual advances, however, homosexual seductive behavior represents an attempt to communicate distress about another problem rather than a genuine search for a sexual partner and should be approached in the same manner.

F. Bizarre sexual behavior such as extremely short miniskirts with high top tennis shoes and gaudy makeup often indicates a severe psychiatric disturbance.

G. Examine the patient for schizophrenia, mania, psychotic depression, drug intoxication or withdrawal, and organic brain syndrome.

REFERENCES

Franks R. Management of the seductive patient. Amer Family Physician 1980; 22:111–114.

Franks R. The angry and seductive patient. In: Simons R, ed. Understanding Human Behavior in Health and Illness. 3rd ed. Baltimore: Williams & Wilkins (in press).

Kardener SH, Feller M, Mensh IN. A survey of physician's attitudes and practices regarding erotic and non-erotic contact with patients. Amer J Psychiatry 1973; 130:1077–1081.

SEDUCTIVE
BEHAVIOR

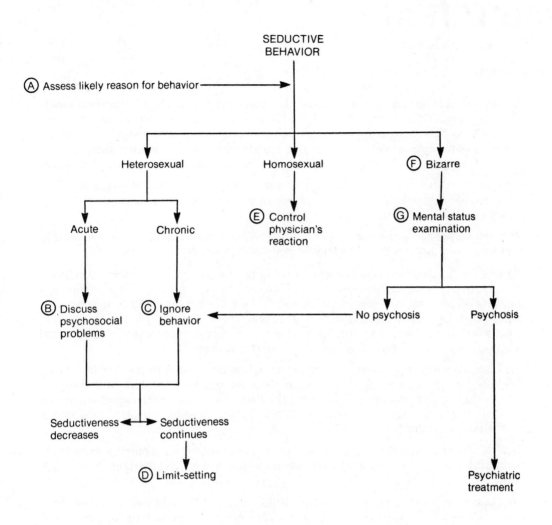

A Assess likely reason for behavior ⟶

Heterosexual

Homosexual

F Bizarre

Acute

Chronic

E Control
physician's
reaction

G Mental status
examination

B Discuss
psychosocial
problems

C Ignore
behavior

No psychosis

Psychosis

Seductiveness
decreases

Seductiveness
continues

D Limit-setting

Psychiatric
treatment

AGITATION

Steven L. Dubovsky, M.D.

COMMENTS

A. A history of recent crises, injuries, illnessess, drug ingestion, and psychiatric treatment should be obtained from the patient and all available informants. Early in the examination, the physician should begin to determine whether agitation has an organic etiology by performing a mental status examination (pp 96–97). A blood screen for psychoactive drugs may be helpful. Care must be taken with any agitated patient to protect both patient and physician.

B. Agitation is the behavioral manifestation of anxiety; the agitated patient is reassured by a calm, confident approach in which the physician displays concern while gently but firmly insisting that the patient remain calm.

C. Restraint may be necessary if the patient does not regain control. Restrained patients must be kept under constant observation while the evaluation proceeds.

D. Patients with organic brain syndromes become agitated when they cannot remember where they are, who important people are, or what is wrong with them (pp 96–97). Agitation in a previously compensated demented patient may be due to a superimposed delirium caused by minor physiologic derangements such as urinary tract infection, dehydration, medication toxicity, or adverse drug interaction. Social or sensory isolation, changes in environment, and recent losses may also produce agitation in demented patients.

E. Antihistamines (e.g., hydroxyzine 50 mg IM or 100 mg orally) may be effective in sedating delirious patients for an EEG; they do not affect the tracing. Low doses (0.5–5 mg) of haloperidol decrease agitation. This drug may be given IV to tranquilize an agitated delirious patient in an emergency. Propranolol (80–320 mg/day) may ameliorate unpredictable violent outbursts in demented patients.

F. Slow IV administration of haloperidol, or, if intracranial pressure is not raised, a short-acting barbiturate may be used to calm agitated patients whose diagnosis is uncertain. Paraldehyde orally or IM is effective.

G. Intoxication with CNS stimulants, cocaine, hallucinogens, PCP, and anticholinergic drugs causes characteristic syndromes that are frequently accompanied by agitation and assaultiveness. Diagnosis and treatment which involves isolation from all but the most calming environmental stimuli and, in some cases, minor tranquilizers are summarized on pp 104–105.

H. Some advocate rapid intramuscular tranquilization of severely agitated manic or schizophrenic patients with nonsedating neuroleptics such as haloperidol (1–5 mg every 30–60 mins) until the patient is sedated. Recent evidence suggests that standard schedules are just as effective. Neuroleptics such as thiothixine and thioridazine may decrease agitation in severely depressed patients.

I. Patients with limited psychological resources or an habitual tendency to become violent when upset often have borderline, histrionic, or antisocial personality disorders. Agitation and assaultiveness in reaction to stress often abate when the patient is told firmly to stop behaving in such a manner. If hospitalization is necessary, an attempt should be made to set a discharge date in advance in order to avoid the development of intense, dependent relationships with staff and other patients that may complicate later discharge. Low doses of antianxiety drugs or haloperidol may be useful acutely, but sedating antipsychotic drugs may cloud the patient's thinking and further reduce his ability to deal with emotional conflict.

J. Rarely, severely excited catatonic patients may need emergency ECT or anesthesia to prevent exhaustion, rhabdomyolysis, and death. ECT is the treatment of choice for depressed

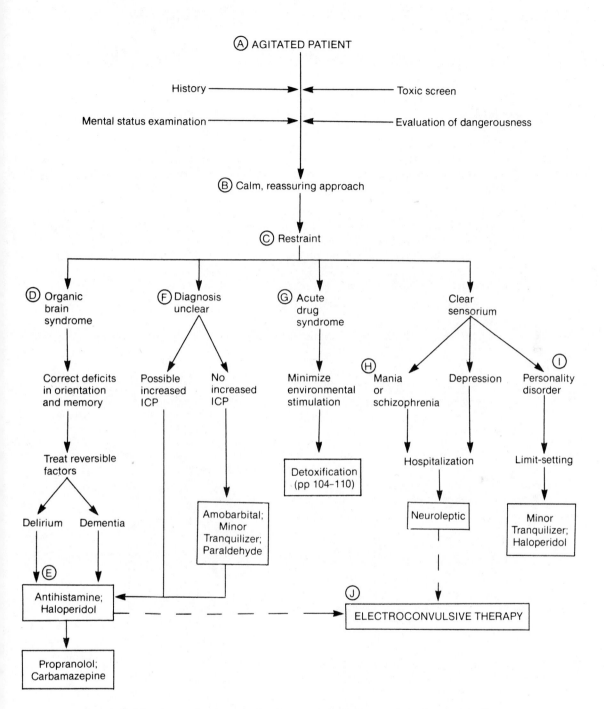

Ⓐ AGITATED PATIENT

History ──────────►│◄────────── Toxic screen

Mental status examination ──────────►│◄────────── Evaluation of dangerousness

Ⓑ Calm, reassuring approach

Ⓒ Restraint

Ⓓ Organic brain syndrome

Ⓕ Diagnosis unclear

Ⓖ Acute drug syndrome

Clear sensorium

Correct deficits in orientation and memory

Possible increased ICP

No increased ICP

Minimize environmental stimulation

Ⓗ Mania or schizophrenia

Depression

Ⓘ Personality disorder

Treat reversible factors

Detoxification (pp 104–110)

Hospitalization

Limit-setting

Delirium   Dementia

Amobarbital; Minor Tranquilizer; Paraldehyde

Neuroleptic

Minor Tranquilizer; Haloperidol

Ⓔ Antihistamine; Haloperidol

Ⓙ ELECTROCONVULSIVE THERAPY

Propranolol; Carbamazepine

patients who do not respond to medication or are too ill to wait for it to take effect. A small number of ECTs may reverse severe agitated deliria when other methods are ineffective.

REFERENCES

Dubovsky SL, Weissberg MP. Clinical Psychiatry in Primary Care. 2nd ed. Baltimore: Williams & Wilkins, 1982.
Shader RI, ed. Manual of Psychiatric Therapeutics. Boston: Little, Brown, 1976.
Slaby AE, Lieb J, Tancredi LR. Handbook of Psychiatric Emergencies. New York: Medical Examination Publishing Co, 1975.

MEDICAL MANAGEMENT OF SUICIDE ATTEMPT BY OVERDOSE

Peter Parks, M.D.

COMMENTS

A. Psychiatrists and other physicians frequently must institute or direct emergency treatment of patients who have attempted suicide by overdose. More than 50% of these individuals have obtained the medication in one prescription from their primary physicians, who did not realize they were suicidal.

B. The circumstances of the attempt, type, and amount of medication ingested, time of ingestion, recent alcohol intake, associated medical problems, reasons for and expectations of the attempt, should be ascertained from the patient and other informants. Toxicology reports may reveal that the patient has ingested unsuspected substances; blood levels may be useful in following response to therapy. Ongoing risk (pp 18–19) must be assessed prior to discharge from the emergency room or hospital.

C. Basic life support should be instituted immediately, and advanced life support as quickly as possible, if the patient does not respond to attempts to arouse him, does not breathe spontaneously, and is pulseless. The patient should then be transferred to an intensive care unit for definitive treatment.

D. Ipecac may remove the ingested drug if gastric emptying has not occurred to a significant degree. The usual adult dose is 30 cc. Because of the danger of aspiration, ipecac should not be administered if the gag reflex is depressed. If more than 30 minutes have elapsed since ingestion, ipecac is unlikely to be successful and may prevent retention of magnesium sulfate and charcoal.

E. If the patient does not have a gag reflex, is seen more than 30 minutes after ingestion, or does not vomit within 15–20 minutes of being given ipecac, lavage with normal saline should be performed, and an attempt should be made to remove pill fragments through a no. 28 nasogastric tube.

F. Magnesium sulfate (200 mg/kg) is used as a purgative to speed the passage of the ingested substance through the GI tract and decrease absorption. Powdered charcoal (1 g/kg) adsorbs the ingested drug, decreasing GI absorption. An experienced clinician should manage life-threatening complications that may not appear immediately after ingestion. The local poison center or Poisondex, a microfilm service offering up-to-date information about ingested substances, can provide necessary toxicological information.

REFERENCES

Krupp MA, Chatton MJ. Current Medical Diagnosis and Treatment. Los Altos, California: Lange Medical Publications, 1982: 961–987.
Rumak BH. Poisondex. National Center for Poison Information, Denver, CO.
Swartz GR. Poisonings. In: Principles and Practice of Emergency Medicine. Philadelphia: WB Saunders, 1978: 1428–1437.

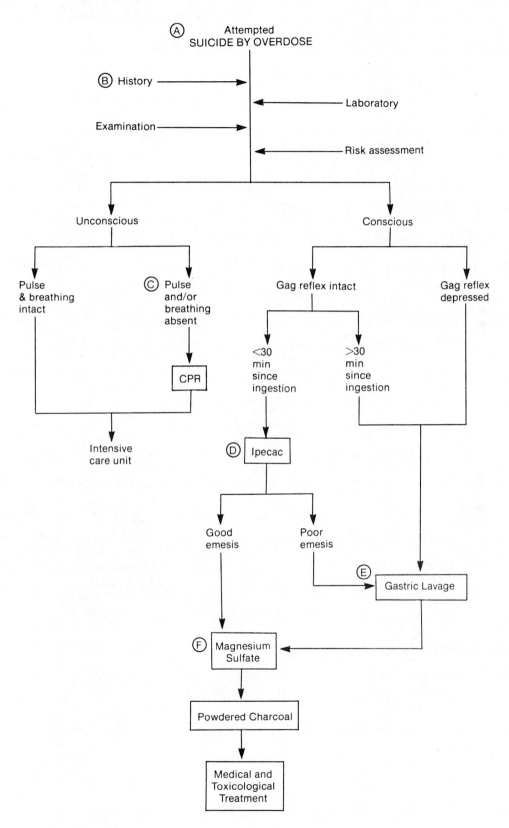

(A) Attempted
SUICIDE BY OVERDOSE

(B) History

Laboratory

Examination

Risk assessment

Unconscious

Conscious

Pulse
& breathing
intact

(C) Pulse
and/or
breathing
absent

Gag reflex intact

Gag reflex
depressed

CPR

<30
min
since
ingestion

>30
min
since
ingestion

Intensive
care unit

(D) Ipecac

Good
emesis

Poor
emesis

(E) Gastric Lavage

(F) Magnesium
Sulfate

Powdered Charcoal

Medical and
Toxicological
Treatment

PSYCHOLOGICAL MANAGEMENT OF ATTEMPTED SUICIDE

Alan Feiger, M.D.

COMMENTS

A. The ongoing risk following a suicide attempt is high if the patient continues to want to die, if the crisis that precipitated the attempt has not been resolved, and if the patient has an ongoing plan that can be carried out. Risk is also increased by communication of intent, hopelessness, chronic or terminal physical illness, a past history of suicide attempts, especially if 3 or more attempts have been made or if these were violent or carefully planned, and a family history of suicide. The majority of patients who commit suicide are depressed and/or alcoholic. Risk is also increased in patients with organic brain syndromes, schizophrenics, and drug abusers. Family members may be important allies or they may covertly or openly encourage suicidal behavior in the patient.

B. Low lethality attempts are characterized by low risk and high chance of rescue, as exemplified by small overdoses and minor lacerations in the presence of a potential rescuer. If supportive family members and friends are available and the patient no longer feels suicidal, especially if the crisis that precipitated the event is resolving, the patient can be discharged from the emergency room and encouraged to seek outpatient treatment. However, only 50% of patients follow through with outpatient therapy. Compliance is increased if an appointment is made within 72 hours with a therapist known personally to the referring physician. Follow-up may be facilitated if the referring doctor actually makes the first appointment for the patient.

C. More serious overdoses, stab wounds, jumps from less than 30 feet, and attempts that do not take place with a rescuer immediately present convey higher lethality. When the patient has made an attempt of moderate lethality, suicidal thoughts without specific plans continue, or an acute, treatable psychiatric disorder is present, close follow-up is warranted to monitor increasing risk and institute intensive treatment. An outpatient appointment should be scheduled for the next day and family members instructed to watch the patient closely.

D. Immediate hospitalization should be considered when a suicide attempt has not resulted in resolution of a crisis, when the patient denies the seriousness of the problem or is unwilling to agree to outpatient treatment, when important people in the patient's life are unsupportive or hostile, or risk is undetermined. Hospitalization is mandatory after a highly dangerous or bizarre suicide attempt, especially if planned so that rescue would not be immediate, even if the patient says that he is no longer suicidal.

E. If suicide potential remains high after the patient is admitted, he must be observed closely and restrained or sedated if necessary. ECT is an option if the patient does not improve quickly.

REFERENCES

Weissman MM. The epidemiology of suicide attempts: 1960–1971. Arch Gen Psychiatry 1974; 30:737–746.

Kaplan HI, Sadock BJ. Management of suicide. In: Modern Synopsis of Psychiatry III. Baltimore: Williams & Wilkins, 1981:706.

Guggenheim FG. Suicide. In: Hackett TP, Cassem NH, eds. Handbook of General Hospital Psychiatry. St. Louis: CV Mosby, 1978:250.

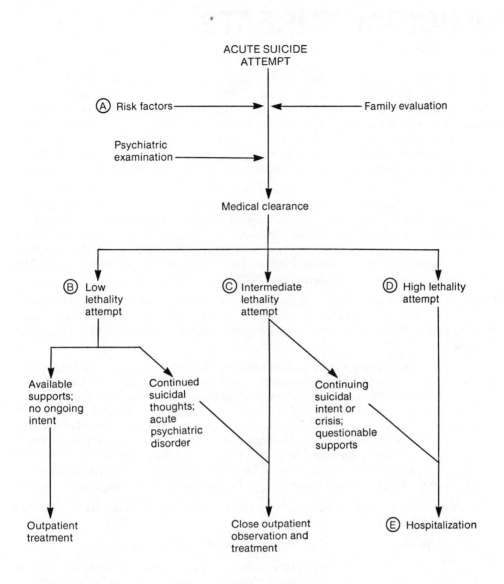

ACUTE SUICIDE
ATTEMPT

(A) Risk factors⟶ ⟵Family evaluation

Psychiatric
examination⟶

Medical clearance

(B) Low
lethality
attempt

(C) Intermediate
lethality
attempt

(D) High lethality
attempt

Available
supports;
no ongoing
intent

Continued
suicidal
thoughts;
acute
psychiatric
disorder

Continuing
suicidal
intent or
crisis;
questionable
supports

Outpatient
treatment

Close outpatient
observation and
treatment

(E) Hospitalization

HOMICIDAL THREATS

Neil Baker, M.D.

A. Immediate high-risk situations often can be identified and defused, even though it is not possible to identify with complete confidence those patients who are not dangerous; long-term dangerousness cannot be predicted. The risk that a patient will act on threats to injure another person is increased in the presence of threats directed against a specific person, definite workable plan, available weapon, history of violence, poor impulse control, organic brain syndrome, intoxication with drugs or alcohol, psychosis, antisocial personality disorder, denial of major problems, family history of violence, and lack of a stable life.

B. The frequency and nature of previous threats and actions, and interventions that have been helpful should be determined. Marital crises, conflicts with authority figures, humiliation, and increased emotional closeness to others commonly precipitate feelings of helplessness that the patient attempts to control with homicidal threats. The threats may arouse in the physician excessive anxiety, helplessness, anger, or denial of the danger, all of which interfere with appropriate therapeutic actions. However, the physician's uneasiness may be the first indication that the patient is dangerous (pp 24–25).

C. The patient may lose control of his impulses in the examining room if he speaks in a loud, threatening voice, uses profanity, paces, glares, is intoxicated or adopts an approach-avoidance posture. The physician's immediate safety should be ensured before proceeding (pp 24–25).

D. Impulse control may be better in the patient without a past history of homicidal threats if the patient does not have a specific or convincing plan, there is no specific victim, threats decrease during the interview, the patient wishes treatment and makes a clear commitment to contact the physician immediately if homicidal feelings increase, and helpful supports are available. If a major psychiatric or medical disorder is present, the patient may be too unpredictable even if he seems calm during the evaluation. The immediate risk is likely to warrant hospitalization if threats continue during the initial interview, if the patient has a specific plan, or if the patient has a significant history of violence. When the clinician believes that a patient presents a clear and immediate danger to another person, he is obligated to warn the potential victim.

E. It is usually safer to hospitalize for further evaluation patients in whom the risk is difficult to assess during the initial evaluation.

F. It is difficult to predict when chronic threats will become acutely dangerous.

G. Hospitalization provides structure, reality testing, impulse control and constructive interactions with other patients. Nonsedating antipsychotic medications can be very useful in controlling acutely agitated patients, but sedatives and antianxiety compounds may decrease internal controls as well as healthy anticipatory anxiety. For both inpatients and outpatients, crisis intervention begins with prohibiting alcohol and drugs, removing available weapons, identifying precipitants, assessing coping skills and bolstering self-esteem. The patient is then helped to view the crisis as an ongoing problem rather than an issue that requires an all-or-nothing immediate solution. Family members and friends should be involved in treatment.

H. When an unwilling patient is coerced into treatment, therapy is likely to produce only unrealistic fantasies of a cure. However, the threatening patient who is distressed by his symptom deserves an active approach. The patient is taught to identify and avoid situations that tend to evoke threats or dangerous behavior. Propranolol, lithium, carbamazepine, and neuroleptics may help some explosive, volatile patients with a history of brain injury, abnormal EEGs, cognitive deficits or emotional lability to gain control of their impulses. If the immediate danger is not too high, the physician should not assume control too quickly in order to ensure that the patient learn to assume as much responsibility for himself as possible.

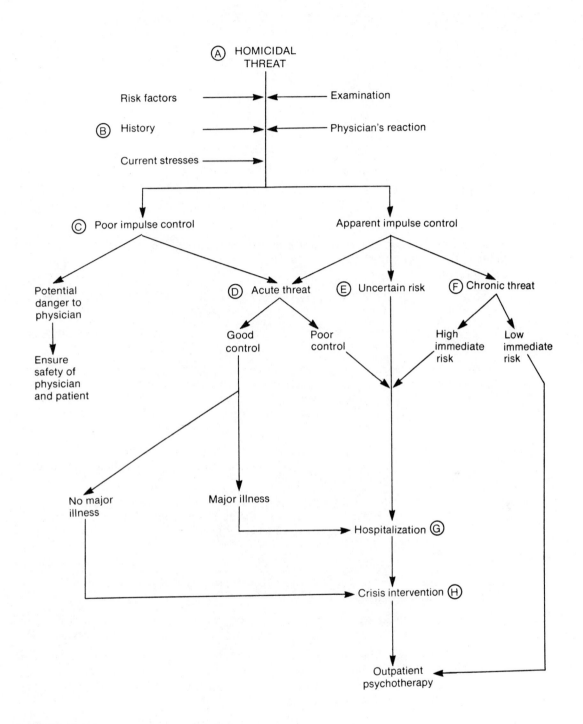

REFERENCES

Monahan J. Clinical prediction of violent behavior. Psychiatric Ann 1982; 12:509–513.

Lion JR, Pasternak SA. Countertransference reactions to violent patients. Amer J Psychiatry 1973; 130:207–210.

Macdonald J. Homicidal Threats. St. Louis: CC Thomas, 1970.

Hallek S. Social violence and aggression. In: Kaplan HI, Freedman AM, Sadock BJ, eds. Comprehensive Textbook of Psychiatry. 3rd ed. Baltimore: Williams & Wilkins, 1980: 3149–3154.

MANAGEMENT OF THE RAPE VICTIM

Ronald D. Franks, M.D.

COMMENTS

A. Although there are no reliable data correlating psychiatric outcome with specific characteristics of the rape, there is no evidence that women consciously or unconsciously invite attack.

B. As with any traumatic event, unresolved or latent psychiatric problems may be precipitated by a rape.

C. The patient's partner may have a strong reaction that he initially denies and that first manifests as a disruption in their relationship.

D. Avoid unnecessarily intrusive questions that may make the patient feel more violated. Ask the patient if she prefers a female physician, and if she would like to have a woman present during the initial examination.

E. Venereal disease must be diagnosed and treated promptly and abortion discussed when appropriate.

F. Short-term use of benzodiazepines is appropriate for severe agitation although they must not replace discussion of the patient's feelings. Since depression also is likely to represent a response to the obvious stress, antidepressants should not be prescribed for the first 3 months unless their use is specifically indicated by a history of depression or by severe vegetative signs (pp 58–59).

G. Patients who become suspicious and fearful of being in situations that recall the rape may benefit from practising biofeedback, hypnosis and other relaxation techniques at times of anxiety and from systematic desensitization.

H. Sexual dysfunctions that were not previously present, which may persist up to 2 years after a rape, may be treated by discussing the way the event has affected the couple's attitudes toward sex and their level of adaptation, and by helping them to reestablish an emotionally intimate relationship.

I. Reexperiencing the rape through discussions and attention to dreams helps the victim to regain a sense of control. The partner, if available, should be involved as a source of support. Self-help groups may also help to relieve feelings of fear and isolation.

J. During regular contact with the patient, in person or by telephone, once a week for 1 to 3 months, encourage but do not pressure the patient to air continuing feelings about the rape.

K. Restricted social activities, sexual problems, insomnia, nightmares, anorexia, depression, suspiciousness, fear of being alone, somatic complaints, fatigue, and difficulty concentrating persist for up to one year in one-third of patients. Further treatment should be offered if the patient is not substantially improved after 1 year.

L. Failure to improve after 3 months may be due to a psychiatric disorder (often depression) or underlying psychological conflicts that have been precipitated or exacerbated by the stress. If insight-oriented psychotherapy does not resolve emotional conflicts, behavior therapy may help the patient suppress ongoing symptomatology.

M. Indications of the emergence of an underlying psychiatric disorder include prolonged or severe depression or anxiety, psychosis, suicidal plans or attempts, and significant functional deterioration.

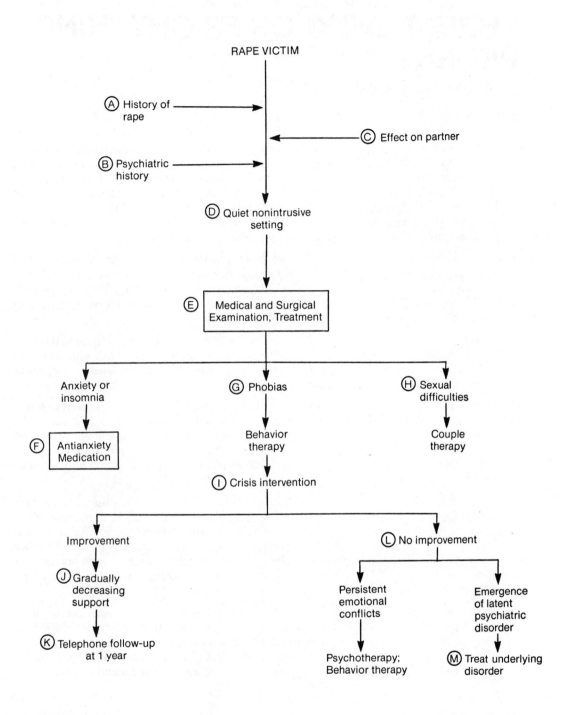

RAPE VICTIM

(A) History of rape

(C) Effect on partner

(B) Psychiatric history

(D) Quiet nonintrusive setting

(E) Medical and Surgical Examination, Treatment

Anxiety or insomnia

(G) Phobias

(H) Sexual difficulties

(F) Antianxiety Medication

Behavior therapy

Couple therapy

(I) Crisis intervention

Improvement

(L) No improvement

(J) Gradually decreasing support

Persistent emotional conflicts

Emergence of latent psychiatric disorder

(K) Telephone follow-up at 1 year

Psychotherapy; Behavior therapy

(M) Treat underlying disorder

REFERENCES

Burgess AW, Holmstrom LD. Adaptive strategies and recovery from rape. Amer J Psychiatry 1979; 136:1278–1282.

Hilberman E. The Rape Victim. New York: Basic Books, 1976.

Burgess AW, Holmstrom LL. Rape: Crisis and Recovery. Bowie, Maryland: Robert J. Brady Co, 1979.

Nadelson CC, Malkah TN, Fackson H, Gormick J. A follow-up study of rape victims. Amer J Psychiatry 1982; 139:1114–1118.

THREATENING OR FRIGHTENING PATIENT

Steven L. Dubovsky, M.D.

COMMENTS

A. A surprising number of patients visit the physician's office or the emergency room carrying some kind of weapon. Every patient who has been injured in a fight, has a threatening manner, or makes the physician uneasy should be asked if he or she is armed. The examiner's discomfort may be the first indication that an apparently calm patient is barely in control of his impulses. Attempts to suppress fear by minimizing the danger, or overestimating the risk, interfere with adequate assessment. History and examination for illness often must be deferred until the safety of patient and physician can be assured.

B. The patient who is allowed to keep his weapon is likely to doubt that the physician will be able to control his murderous impulses and may attempt to force others to limit his behavior by escalating it. If the patient does not surrender his weapon immediately, the danger is likely to be high and assistance should be sought at once. The physician should leave the examining room until the patient is disarmed.

C. Factors associated with high immediate risk of dangerous behavior, in addition to those on p 20, include: intrusion on the examiner's "body space"; psychosis, especially with command hallucinations (voices instructing the patient to hurt someone); and absence of supportive people who might prevent the dangerous behavior.

D. Even if the high-risk patient is not agitated, the physician should not proceed unless a sufficient number of other personnel is available to subdue him safely if necessary. The patient is reassured and becomes less threatening when he knows that he will not be allowed to injure anyone; his self-esteem is bolstered when he is considered important enough to command a strong show of force. If help is not available, the patient should be allowed to leave the doctor's office.

E. If the patient becomes agitated or continues to threaten, he should be offered medication (pp 14–15) orally first. Restraint may be necessary if medication may be dangerous, if the patient refuses it, or if the situation is urgent. One person should be responsible for each of the patient's extremities and one for his head, as one extremity at a time is placed in leather restraints. The restrained patient should be kept under constant observation to prevent him from strangling himself or getting loose and to monitor for prolonged struggling that can lead to myoglobinuria.

F. After evaluating for organic brain syndrome, the physician should assess: precipitating events; provocations; history of antisocial, threatening or assaultive behavior; availability of weapon; psychotic symptoms, especially command hallucinations; history and family history of psychosis; homicidal and/or suicidal thoughts; alcohol and drug use; available supports; spouse and/or child abuse; head injury; neurological disease in patient and family.

REFERENCES

Dietz PE, Rodaw RT. Risks and benefits of working with violent patients. Psychiatric Ann 1982; 5:502–508.
Shader RI. Manual of Psychiatric Emergencies. Boston: Little, Brown, 1975.
Weissberg MP, Dubovsky SL. Assessment of psychiatric emergencies in medical practice. Primary Care 1977; 4:651–656.

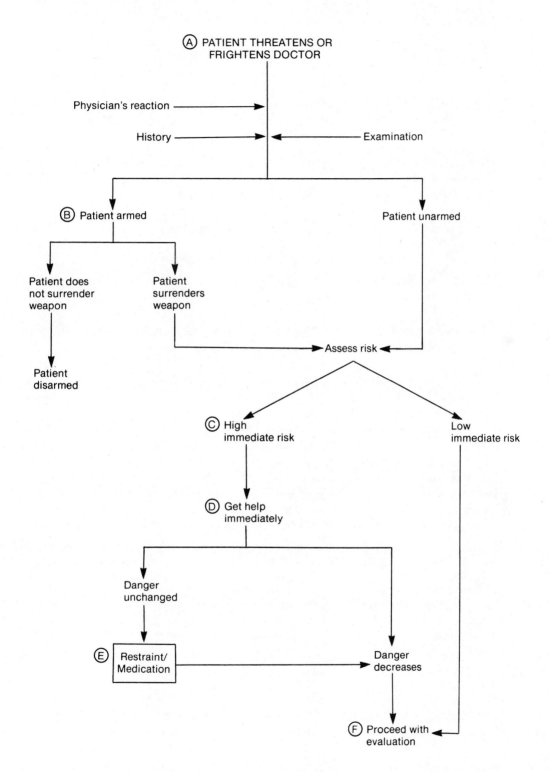

SPOUSE ABUSE

Marjorie W. Leidig, Ph.D.

COMMENTS

A. Women are much more likely than men to be injured by a partner. Physical abuse occurs at all socioeconomic levels, and often is detected first by the family physician, emergency physician, or gynecologist. Suspicious physical findings in the outpatient include bruises, black eyes, and abdominal, shoulder, or back pain. Fractures and bleeding may require hospitalization. Patients may delay seeking attention and conceal the actual cause of injury. Psychological symptoms associated with abuse include chronic marital problems, low self-esteem, self-blame, anxiety, agitation, paranoia, requests for medication, and vague thoughts of suicide.

B. Baseline data include the overall pattern of abuse, its duration and intensity, and available resources. Alcohol abuse may be invoked to "justify" battering; however, alcoholism is no more likely to be a cause of battering than is any other stress.

C. Impatience with the victim's sense of helplessness, assumptions that she precipitates abuse or remains in the relationship because she is masochistic, and uncontrollable anger at the batterer, may interfere with treatment.

D. The patient is likely to reveal and discuss the problem if she is made to feel safe, is not criticized, and is assured of confidentiality.

E. Psychotropic drugs other than short-term analgesics are generally considered countertherapeutic to the psychological task the patient must accomplish. A female therapist is more likely to understand the patient's dilemma, and is a better source of identification for the patient. Books about battering are helpful because they teach the patient that she is not alone, they describe potential sources of help, and they enable the patient to see herself as a "battered woman", which helps decrease passivity and mobilize anger and a wish for help.

F. A few episodes of abuse that do not cause major physical injury, especially if the patient affirms that she will leave if abuse is ever repeated, convey relatively low risk. Intermediate-risk situations result in more serious trauma and occur once a month to once every 3 months; feelings of helplessness, anxiety, and depression are more prominent. Chronic, potentially lethal incidents indicate high risk requiring immediate hospitalization to protect the patient.

G. The most important curative factor is a therapist familiar with the treatment of battered women. Psychotherapy should address the reasons why the patient remains in an abusive situation, including fear, economic dependency, lack of supports, and inability to trust her own perceptions because she has become isolated from usual sources of concensual validation. She is likely to have had family training in seeing men as strong and powerful and women as acquiescent, weak, and nurturing. She is likely to have difficulty dealing with her anger; role modeling by the therapist of appropriate assertiveness and expression of anger is helpful.

H. Separate treatment for the partner and couples therapy may help to resolve acute problems that are being expressed in battering, the man often drops out after a few sessions, especially if he is reassured that his wife will not leave him. Individual treatment for the batterer is often ineffective because he will not take responsibility for the problem or does not keep appointments. Victim support groups with trained group leaders may accomplish the same goal as individual treatment.

I. A safe-house protects the patient, introduces her to other battered women, and provides immediate, helpful advice and experience of alternative living arrangements. A restraining order, filing assault charges, or initiation of divorce require legal assistance.

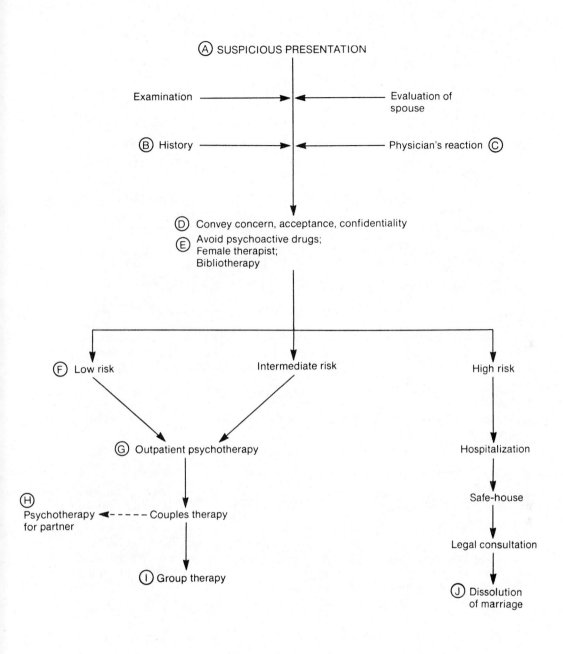

A SUSPICIOUS PRESENTATION

Examination ⟶ ⟵ Evaluation of spouse

B History ⟶ ⟵ Physician's reaction C

D Convey concern, acceptance, confidentiality

E Avoid psychoactive drugs;
Female therapist;
Bibliotherapy

F Low risk   Intermediate risk   High risk

G Outpatient psychotherapy   Hospitalization

H
Psychotherapy ⟵ ----- Couples therapy   Safe-house
for partner

                                              Legal consultation

I Group therapy   J Dissolution
                                                of marriage

J. The physician should recommend immediate separation to protect both partners in high-risk
    situations.

CHARACTERISTICS OF SOME PSYCHOSES

Neil Baker, M.D., Deborah A. Coyle, M.D.

COMMENTS

A. The current diagnostic nomenclature (DSM-3) specifies that symptoms must be continuously present for at least 6 months to diagnose schizophrenia. If symptoms last <6 months, a schizophreniform disorder is said to be present.

B. Mania may be extremely difficult to differentiate from schizophrenia. Good premorbid functioning, remission of symptoms, and family history of affective disorders but not schizophrenia can be more reliable than presenting symptoms in identifying mania.

C. Schizoaffective disorder is the only condition that is not defined in DSM-3. This disorder may be present if the examiner cannot determine whether schizophrenia or mania is present.

D. Brief reactive psychosis lasts <2 weeks and usually occurs in patients with borderline personality disorder in reaction to a severe stress, drug abuse, or a problem in the doctor-patient relationship.

E. Better premorbid work and marital and social functioning suggest that an affective component (depression or mania) may be present, no matter how severe presenting symptoms may be. The therapeutic implication is that an antidepressant or lithium might appropriately be added.

F. Prognosis for recovery of premorbid functioning is better (1) if psychosis represents a response to a clear precipitating stress, and (2) in affective disorders, brief reactive psychoses, and schizophreniform psychoses.

G. Although many manic patients recover completely from acute episodes, 20–35% have a chronic course.

H. Treatment of acute schizophrenia requires at least 300 mg/day of chlorpromazine or its equivalent in high-potency (nonsedating) neuroleptics. Chronic treatment requires 75 mg/day (pp 179).

I. Not all manic patients respond to lithium. Carbamazepam, propranolol, clonidine, ECT, and perhaps calcium-antagonists are possible alternatives. Neuroleptics are often necessary until lithium becomes effective, but haloperidol or thioridazine combined with lithium may cause severe neurological syndromes (pp 179).

REFERENCES

American Psychiatric Association: Diagnostic and Statistical Manual of Mental Disorders. 3rd ed. Washington, DC: APA Press, 1980.
Pope HG, Lipinski JF. Diagnosis in schizophrenia and manic-depressive illness. Arch Gen Psychiatry 1978; 35:811–828.

CHARACTERISTICS OF SOME PSYCHOSES

	Age and Mode of Onset	Premorbid Ⓔ Functioning	Presenting Features	Course	Prognosis Ⓕ	Drug Treatment
Schizophrenia Ⓐ	Teens–twenties Insidious onset	Poor	Withdrawal Delusions of control Mood–incongruent delusions	Deteriorating	Poor	Neuroleptic Ⓗ
Schizophreniform disorder	<45 Variable onset	Fair	Like schizophrenia	Remitting	Good	Neuroleptic Lithium
Mania Ⓑ	Usually <30 Acute onset	Good	Hyperactivity Irritability Delusions of wealth, power, grandeur	Episodic; 50–75% chance of recurrence	Good Ⓖ	Neuroleptic Ⓘ plus lithium
Psychotic depression	Any age Acute onset	Good	Withdrawal Agitation Delusions of disease, decay, punishment	Epidosic; 50% chance of recurrence	Good	Neuroleptic plus anti-depressant or ECT
Schizoaffective Ⓒ disorder	Probably <45 Variable onset	Variable	Schizophrenic and affective symptoms	Variable; may be chronic	Variable	Neuroleptic plus anti-depressant or lithium
Brief reactive Ⓓ psychosis	Teens–early 30s Acute onset	Good	Paranoia Hostility	Short-lived	Good	Nonsedating neuroleptic
Paranoid Disorder	Probably mid 30s – mid 40s	Good	Thinking intact except for circumscribed delusional concern	Acute	Good	Nonsedating neuroleptic
Delirium	Any age, especially older Acute onset No past psychiatric disturbance	Good	Confusion Fluctuating level of consciousness; Concrete delusions derived from real-life events	Depends on underlying illness	Good short-term, increased long-term morbidity	Nonsedating neuroleptic

ACUTE PSYCHOSIS

Neil Baker, M.D. and Alan Feiger, M.D.

COMMENTS

A. Acute psychosis is a nonspecific symptom complex that includes delusions, hallucinations, severe disorganization, incoherent thinking and loss of reality testing, that may be caused by a number of functional or organic disorders. Initial history should explore medical illnesses and treatments, use of alcohol and drugs, level of premorbid functioning, psychiatric history, family history and recent stresses. Since the patient is likely to be uncooperative or unreliable, additional information should be obtained from family members, friends, previous physicians and therapists, other referral sources, and police when appropriate. Exacerbation or reemergence of previously controlled psychotic symptoms is likely to be due to discontinuation of therapy, a psychosocial crisis, or drug or alcohol ingestion.

B. Lack of cooperation, poor attention, hallucinations, and delusions complicate mental status testing for organic brain disease in the psychotic patient. However, a first episode of acute psychosis after age 45, visual, gustatory and olfactory hallucinations, focal neurological signs, motor perseveration, dysarthria, ataxia, and nystagmus suggest that psychosis has an organic cause. Amphetamines, cocaine, hallucinogens, and PCP may produce paranoid psychoses in the presence of a clear sensorium (pp 112–113).

C. Psychotic patients often evoke fear, discomfort and anger; the physician may then omit portions of the examination in an attempt to increase emotional distance from the patient.

D. If the patient interprets portions of the examination in a bizarre, sexualized or aggressive manner, the procedure should be explained carefully, and questions answered truthfully. All procedures should occur within the patient's view. Frightening or symbolic examinations (pelvic, rectal exam) may be deferred, but no *necessary* procedures should be delayed.

E. Features of hospitalization that are helpful to these patients include: a consistent and predictable environment; limits set on destructive behavior by the patient or significant others; crisis intervention to identify precipitating stresses, help the patient gain insight into his decompensation, and modify pathogenic situations; and family therapy to resolve conflicts. Behavioral approaches and psychosocial interventions effective in the past should be reinstituted.

F. Restrained or secluded patients should be allowed to regain control gradually.

G. A brief explanation of the motivation underlying his behavior may help the patient regain control. Inform him firmly about behaviors that are unacceptable. Restriction of visitors may be necessary.

H. If the diagnosis is unclear and no medication is required, a brief period of observation is indicated. Rapid remission suggests a brief reactive psychosis (pp 28–29), and early discharge is indicated. Nonsedating neuroleptics may be helpful short-term; avoid sedating and addictive drugs. Abrupt worsening of psychotic symptoms 12 to 72 hours after admission suggests an abstinence syndrome (pp 106–107).

REFERENCES

Klein DF, Gittelman R, Quitkin F, Rifkin A. Clinical Management of the Various Stages and Subtypes of Schizophrenia. In: Diagnosis and Drug Treatment of Psychiatric Disorders: Adults and Children. Baltimore: Williams & Wilkins, 1980; 145.

May PRA. Treatment of Schizophrenia. New York: Science House, 1968.

Kessler KA, Waletzky JP. Clinical use of the antipsychotics. Amer J Psychiatry 1981; 138:2.

Pincus J, Tucker GJ. Behavioral Neurology. New York: Oxford Press, 1978: 80–120.

Walker JI, Brodie HKH. Paranoid disorders. In: Kaplan HI, Freedman AM, Sadock BJ. Comprehensive Textbook of Psychiatry. 3rd ed. Baltimore: Williams & Wilkins, 1980: 1288–1299.

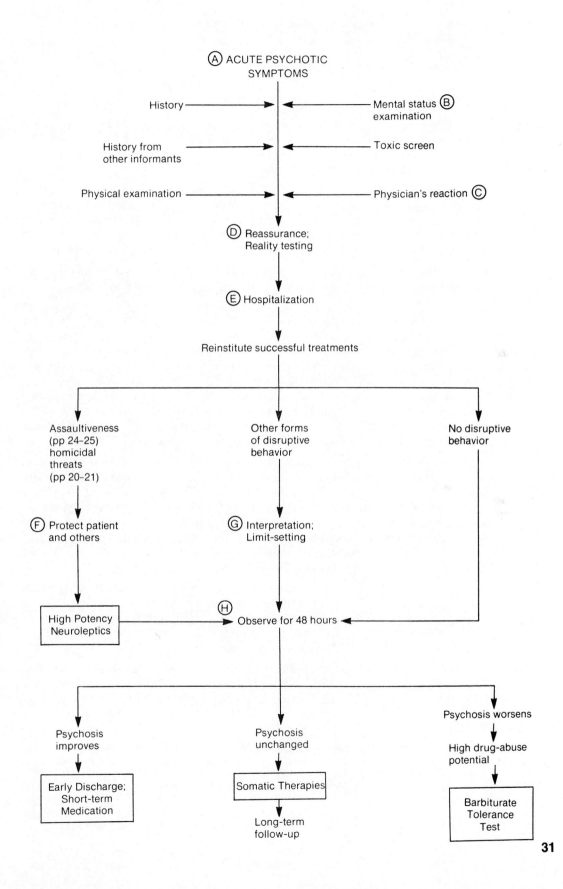

A ACUTE PSYCHOTIC
SYMPTOMS

History ⟶ ⟵ Mental status B
examination

History from ⟶ ⟵ Toxic screen
other informants

Physical examination ⟶ ⟵ Physician's reaction C

D Reassurance;
Reality testing

E Hospitalization

Reinstitute successful treatments

Assaultiveness   Other forms   No disruptive
(pp 24–25)   of disruptive   behavior
homicidal   behavior
threats
(pp 20–21)

F Protect patient   G Interpretation;
and others   Limit-setting

High Potency   H
Neuroleptics   Observe for 48 hours ⟵

Psychosis   Psychosis   Psychosis worsens
improves   unchanged

                                                    High drug-abuse
                                                    potential

Early Discharge;   Somatic Therapies   Barbiturate
Short-term   Tolerance
Medication   Long-term   Test
                                 follow-up

ATYPICAL PSYCHOSES

Neil Baker, M.D.

COMMENTS

A. This chapter addresses psychoses with mixtures of schizophrenic and affective symptoms such as schizoaffective and schizophreniform disorders and major affective disorders with mood incongruent delusions or hallucinations. Specialized treatments in addition to standard approaches (pp 30–31) are summarized.

B. Features suggesting organic brain syndrome (pp 96–97) require a thorough medical evaluation. A few unreplicated studies suggest that some episodic psychoses are associated with dysrrhythmias in the limbic system, oneiroid states with disorders of glucose metabolism, and periodic catatonia with abnormalities of nitrogen balance, urinary catecholamines and serum cholesterol.

C. When symptoms are unusual and confusing, the physician may attempt to fit them into familiar diagnostic categories or may attempt multiple uncoordinated interventions.

D. Although episodic and recurrent psychoses are not nosologically distinct from other atypical psychoses, they are more likely to respond to lithium and/or anticonvulsants. Atypical cycloid psychoses resemble manic depressive psychoses and respond to lithium and ECT; however, familial patterns may be different, elated states may be associated more with tranquility than irritability, and the prognosis may be better. Epileptiform abnormalities in the limbic system in episodic psychoses are suggested by confusion, precipitous onset, intermittent course with symptom-free intervals, soft neurological signs, partial amnesia for psychosis and abnormal EEG. Periodic catatonia is a rare disorder characterized by episodes of excitement or stupor with abrupt onset and cessation. In addition to neuroleptics and lithium, some psychiatrists have reported some success with large doses of thyroxine.

E. Some atypical psychoses result in a generalized disturbance in functioning. Oneiroid states are characterized by dreamlike perceptual distortions with hallucinations in multiple sensory modalities. Some patients respond to treatment for schizophrenia, and others to treatment for schizoaffective disorder. Brief psychoses that occur without a precipitating stress are otherwise similar to brief reactive psychoses (pp 28–29) but may differ with respect to family history. Treatment of the two conditions is the same. The course, outcome and treatment of late-onset paraphrenia are identical to schizophrenia, but the onset is after age 45 and paranoia tends to be more prominent.

F. Atypical psychoses with persistent delusions or hallucinations in only one area, especially hypochondriacal delusions, are not associated with other signs of thought disorder. Premorbid adjustment generally is good, although considerable anxiety or paranoia may accompany the delusion. Symptoms may be acute or chronic. If neuroleptics and other standard approaches to psychosis are ineffective, pimozide may help.

G. Long-term follow-up of unusual syndromes is essential to ensure that atypical presentations of more common disorders, especially organic brain syndromes, have not been overlooked. Ongoing psychosocial care is similar to that for other psychotic patients.

REFERENCES

Monroe RR. DSM-3 style diagnoses of the episodic disorders. J Nerv Ment Dis 1982; 11:664.
Lesser IM. Unusual presentations of schizophrenia. In: Friedmann CTH, Faguet RA, eds. Extraordinary Disorders of Human Behavior. New York, London: Plenum Press, 1982: 293.
Munroe A. Monosymptomatic hypochondriacal psychosis: new aspects of an old syndrome. J Psychiatr Treat Eval 1980; 2:79.
Lehmann HE. Schizophrenia: clinical features. In: Kaplan HI, Freedman AM, Sadoch BJ, eds. Comprehensive Textbook of Psychiatry. 3rd ed. Baltimore: Williams & Wilkins, 1980: 1171.

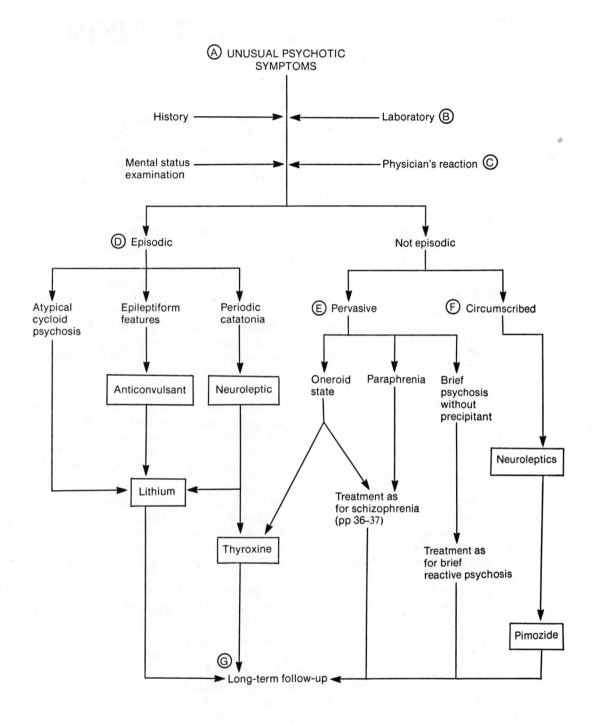

BIZARRE OR UNUSUAL THINKING

Neil Baker, M.D.

COMMENTS

A. The histories of patients whose thoughts are bizarre, unusual, or inappropriate may be difficult to clarify without contacting other informants. Psychiatric and medical history, drug and alcohol use, recent stresses, hallucinations, suspiciousness, delusions, legal problems, and signs of organic brain disease should be examined. Odd thoughts become delusional when they are fixed, false beliefs out of keeping with the patient's cultural or religious background that cannot be corrected by an appeal to logic.

B. The possibility of physical factors affecting the patient's thoughts is increased by an acute personality change with good premorbid functioning, negative psychiatric history, recent illness or injury, and signs of organic brain disease on mental status examination. Intoxication and withdrawal commonly produce abnormal thought processes.

C. Psychosis is suggested by loose associations, incoherence, hallucinations, delusions, markedly inappropriate or bizarre affect or behavior, lack of awareness of irrationality, and pervasive or disabling symptoms. Suspiciousness leads many paranoid patients to conceal some portion of their thinking. Treatment of the psychotic patient should be instituted on an inpatient basis (pp 30–31). When the diagnosis is unclear, extended outpatient follow-up is indicated. Obtain projective psychological tests and an MMPI (pp 176–177). If psychosis is strongly suspected or a psychosocial crisis is present, evaluation should take place in the hospital.

D. Malingerers may consciously behave in an unusual manner in order to obtain some clear-cut external goal. Patients with factitious disorders simulate mental illness for reasons outside of their awareness. Symptoms usually reflect a conscious or unconscious notion of the manifestations of psychosis. The voluntary nature of fabricated symptoms should be discussed with the patient in a manner that avoids needless humiliation. The more acute the disorder, the more amenable the patient is likely to be.

E. Unusual thinking, a common chronic feature of schizotypal and paranoid personality disorders, may become more pronounced with stress; patients with histrionic, borderline and narcissistic personalities tend to display dramatic or distorted cognitive processes in the context of generally intact thinking. The rituals of compulsive patients and the suspiciousness and projection of sociopathic patients are odd although not psychotic. Patients with personality disorders have inflexible approaches to the environment; they find it difficult to adapt to change. Focusing on unusual thinking with such patients may result in an increase in bizarre thoughts in order to gain the physician's attention and to avoid problem solving. Identify current stresses, clarify the patient's reaction, and encourage the patient to resolve conflicts.

F. Disorganization and disordered thinking in patients with personality disorders can be minimized by adapting the physician's approach to the specific needs of the patient. In treating schizoid and paranoid patients keep meetings brief, avoid excessive friendliness, and do not expect them to discuss emotions or intimate details. Set limits on the destructive behavior and unrealistic expectations of borderline and narcissistic patients. Compulsive patients may be reassured by detailed explanations of the illness and its treatment and by involving them in treatment decisions.

G. Low self-esteem, apathy and notions of poverty or illness in depressed patients, and grandiosity and racing thoughts in manics may yield confusing histories.

H. Residual schizophrenia may lead to persistent unusual thinking.

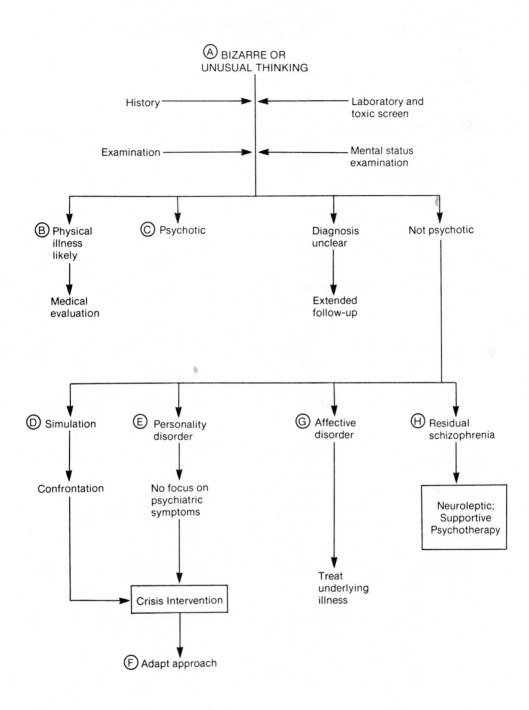

REFERENCES

American Psychiatric Association: Diagnostic and Statistical Manal of Mental Disorders. 3rd ed. Washington, DC: APA, 1980.

Linn L. Clinical manifestations of psychiatric disorders. In: Kaplan HI, Freedman AM, Sadock BJ, eds. Comprehensive Textbook of Psychiatry. 3rd ed. Baltimore: Williams & Wilkins, 1980: 990–1034.

Vaillant GE, Perry JC. Personality disorders. In: Kaplan HI, Freedman AM, Sadock BJ, eds. Comprehensive Textbook of Psychiatry. 3rd ed. Baltimore: Williams & Wilkins, 1980: 1562–1590.

CHRONIC SCHIZOPHRENIA

Alan Feiger, M.D.

COMMENTS

A. Schizophrenia strikes one of every 100 people. Since only 25 percent enjoy a complete recovery, over 1 million Americans need aftercare for chronic schizophrenia. Following discharge from custodial care, many chronic schizophrenics have settled in inner city areas; their concerns about poverty, social isolation, crime, lack of transportation, poor nutritional status, lack of privacy and poor medical care are real. Home visits by a physician or nurse and meetings with caretakers are essential to an evaluation of these stresses. Poor nutritional status and disregard for health and hygiene lead to a high risk of associated physical illness for which only 25 percent of chronic schizophrenics receive adequate care. Careful examination reveals occult medical problems in up to 40 percent of patients.

B. Family involvement is crucial to the success of long-term care. The physician should elicit and correct misconceptions about schizophrenia, particularly that either family or patient are to blame. Symptoms, potential complications, available resources, and support groups should be discussed, including the National Alliance for the Mentally Ill.

C. Psychotherapy should focus on present-problem solving rather than insight into deep-seated conflicts. The patient usually needs help with reality testing, problems in daily living, and morale. Even if he appears withdrawn, his relationship with the physician is likely to be extremely important to him.

D. The relapse rate after 1 year of treatment is more than twice as high for patients taking placebo therapy as for those receiving maintenance antipsychotic medication. The patient should receive the lowest dosage that will prevent relapse.

E. Schizophrenic patients may abuse drugs and alcohol in an attempt at self-medication. Education about adverse effects of such abuse and an increase in dosage of neuroleptic may help.

F. Increasing the dosage of antipsychotic medication may alleviate depression. On the other hand, bradykinesia or other Parkinsonian side effects may mimic depression. Such pseudodepression responds to either lowering antipsychotic dosages or adding antiparkinsonian drugs. Individual psychotherapy or group or family therapy should ease grief over lost abilities. Antidepressants have not been proven efficacious with schizophrenia.

G. Periodic breakthroughs of psychotic behavior and violence may be due to noncompliance, which occurs in 50 percent of schizophrenics, inadequate dosage of neuroleptic, or excessive family demands. Careful documentation and discussion of noncompliance are important. Approximately 25 percent of chronic schizophrenics require long-term care because of continued dangerous behavior or severe disability.

H. Negative symptoms such as demoralization, inflexibility, apathy, ambivalence, and anhedonia respond poorly to medication. Group therapy, self-help groups, assertiveness training, and partial hospitalization may ameliorate social deficits and provide social input.

I. Decreased volition or concentration, over sedation or Parkinson side effects of medication, or high social demands may impair vocational performance. If retraining or job change cannot be arranged, disability payments may be necessary.

REFERENCES

Torrey EF. Surviving Schizophrenia; A Family Manual. New York: Harper & Row, 1983.
Mendel WM. Schizophrenia; The Experience and Its Treatment. San Francisco: Jessey-Bass, 1976.

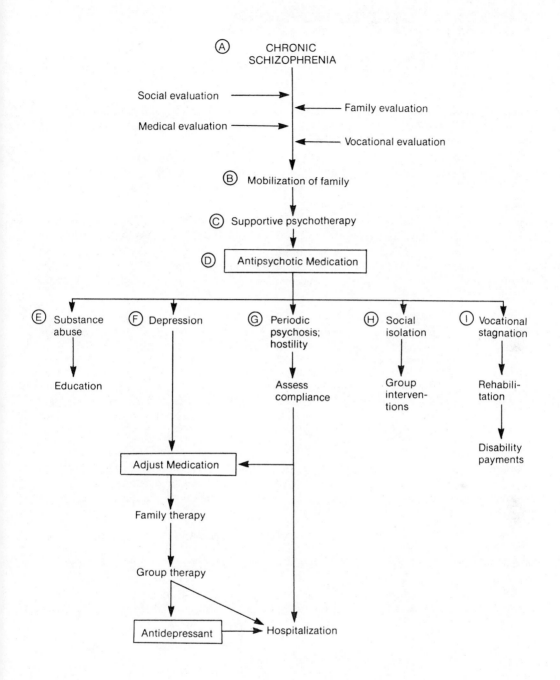

(A) CHRONIC
SCHIZOPHRENIA

Social evaluation ⟶

⟵ Family evaluation

Medical evaluation ⟶

⟵ Vocational evaluation

(B) Mobilization of family

(C) Supportive psychotherapy

(D) Antipsychotic Medication

(E) Substance abuse

(F) Depression

(G) Periodic psychosis; hostility

(H) Social isolation

(I) Vocational stagnation

Education

Assess compliance

Group interventions

Rehabilitation

Disability payments

Adjust Medication

Family therapy

Group therapy

Antidepressant ⟶ Hospitalization

Manos Nikoas, Gkiouzepas J, Logothetis J. The need for continuous use of antiparkinsonian medication with chronic schizophrenic patients receiving long-term neuroleptic therapy. Amer J Psychiatry, 1981; 138:2.

Mendel W. Chronic Schizophrenia: Supportive Care Theory and Technique. Los Angeles: Mara Books, 1975.

Morrison R. Your Brother's Keeper. Chicago: Nelson Hall, 1981.

CHRONIC PSYCHOSIS

Neil Baker, M.D.

COMMENTS

A. This chapter outlines a general approach to chronic psychoses. The patient may not be a reliable historian; obtain additional history from medical records, family, and support services. Determine aspects of treatment or the social environment that maintain stability, events that usually precipitate relapses, signs and symptoms of past decompensations, highest level of functioning, compliance, use of alcohol and drugs, and social service supports. Mental status examination should document chronic abnormalities in order to measure acute changes.

B. The goal of psychotherapy is to help the chronically psychotic patient adapt to everyday demands. The therapist should be active, direct, and hopeful but realistic. Avoid excessive familiarity that might frighten the patient and avoid encouraging more dependency than is necessary. Insight into the limitations imposed by the patient's illness, the patient's feelings about himself and behavior that exacerbates psychoses; however, awareness of deep psychological conflicts is not usually a goal in chronic care.

C. Reduction of environmental stressors is important. Discussions with employers and mobilization of social services may ameliorate pressures that exacerbate psychosis. Decreasing hostility, overinvolvement, or intrusiveness of the family can help stabilize the patient.

D. Antipsychotic drugs decrease relapse rates in schizophrenics (pp 36–37). The risk of tardive dyskinesia may be decreased by the lowest dose that prevents relapse; there is no evidence that drug holidays prevent tardive dyskinesia. Patients with bipolar and schizoaffective disorders may benefit from long-term treatment with lithium and antidepressants. Drug discontinuation may be attempted after the equivalent of several cycles has passed without serious decompensation.

E. Relapse or exacerbation is often caused by noncompliance. Common reasons for noncompliance include distrust of the physician, delusions about the medication, side effects, sabotage of treatment by significant others, a wish to remain psychotic, and financial problems.

F. Loss of a significant relationship can be disorganizing. Reality testing, education about affects normally evoked by loss, and provision of the support that had been supplied by the lost person help restore equilibrium. Problems with finances or living situation often require aggressive interventions with social agencies. Chronically psychotic patients are very sensitive to any change, including changes in the physician's attitude. The physician should tell the patient directly why his attitude has changed and then reestablish the previous mode of interaction.

G. Be alert to symptoms not in the patient's usual repertoire. Medical illnesses and other psychiatric disorders may be overlooked in chronically psychotic patients because the patient cannot communicate symptoms clearly and because all complaints tend to be ascribed to the psychosis.

REFERENCES

Grinspoon L. Psychiatry Update, 1982. Washington, DC: APA, 1982.

Vaugn CE, Leff JP. The influence of family and social factors on the course of psychiatric illness. Br J Psychiatry 1976; 129:125–137.

Lehmann H. Schizophrenia: clinical features. In: Kaplan HI, Freedman AM, Sadock BJ, eds. Comprehensive Textbook of Psychiatry. 3rd ed. Baltimore: Williams & Wilkins, 1980: 1153–1192.

CHRONIC PSYCHOSIS

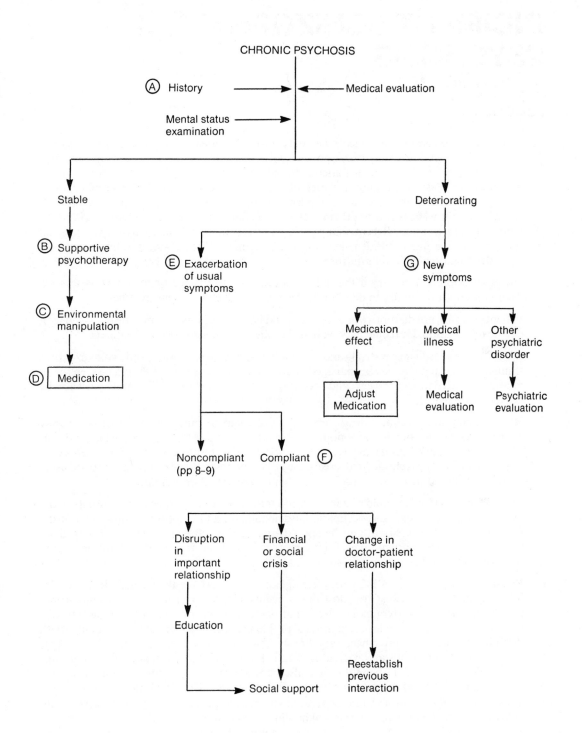

INCIPIENT SCHIZOPHRENIC PSYCHOSIS

Alan Feiger, M.D.

COMMENTS

A. A prodromal phase characterized by anxiety, insomnia, ideas of reference, preoccupation with bodily functions, disorganization, and social withdrawal often precedes frankly psychotic episodes in schizophrenic patients. Rapid initiation of treatment can prevent further deterioration. Past and family histories of psychosis, mode of presentation of previous psychotic episodes, and a detailed description of current symptoms and the patient's thoughts about what is causing them, help to elucidate what may at first appear to be an innocuous presentation. Recent change in level of functioning, availability of psychosocial supports, suicide and homicide risks should be determined. Mental status testing may reveal an underlying organic brain syndrome.

B. Hospitalization is necessary if the patient is a danger to himself or to others, is severely disorganized, or continues to deteriorate despite intensive outpatient treatment.

C. Patients who are not disruptive or dangerous and have intact supports may be managed with day hospitalization. Outcome may be better in these settings for selected patients.

D. If the therapeutic alliance is strong and the family is supportive, tolerant, and avoids excessive stimulation, the patient may be managed as an outpatient. The patient should be seen for 30 minutes at least 3 times per week, and encouraged to call at any time. The family must also be actively involved.

E. High-potency antipsychotic drugs are better tolerated in outpatients than low-potency neuroleptics because of fewer autonomic and sedative effects. Although prophylactic administration of antiparkinsonian drugs is controversial, it may be more justified for patients who are not yet frankly psychotic, to decrease the risk of noncompliance. If such drugs are used, an attempt should be made to discontinue them gradually after 2 months.

F. The patient and family should be educated about the course and suspected biological factors of schizophrenia. Social and occupational demands on and emotional stimulation of the patient should be decreased, and he should be helped to anticipate and deal with daily stresses. Respect the patient's need for interpersonal distance, and avoid exploration of deep psychological conflicts.

G. Rehabilitation, which takes 1–3 years after signs of psychosis have abated, includes maintaining the patient on the lowest drug dose that prevents relapse. The patient must be monitored closely for subtle extrapyramidal effects that decrease responsiveness ("strait-jacketing"), tardive dyskinesia, and unsuspected medical problems. Vocational rehabilitation or help with disability payments are often necessary. Social rehabilitation is facilitated by group therapy, which fosters social skills and decreases isolation and stigmatization, and self-help groups such as Recovery, Inc. The patient should also be advised not to live alone so that social skills can be maintained and the patient's functioning monitored. Concomitant depression, drug abuse and demoralization should be treated vigorously (pp 36–37). Psychotherapy should help the patient acquire a realistic view of his illness while emphasizing all character strengths, signs of improvement and self-control over symptoms. Family therapy and self-help groups such as the National Alliance for the Mentally Ill often provide important support and guidance.

H. Reassessment of diagnosis and treatment is necessary if the patient has not improved significantly after 6 weeks of appropriate therapy. If organic brain syndrome, affective disorder, personality disorder and factitious disorder are carefully excluded, noncompliance

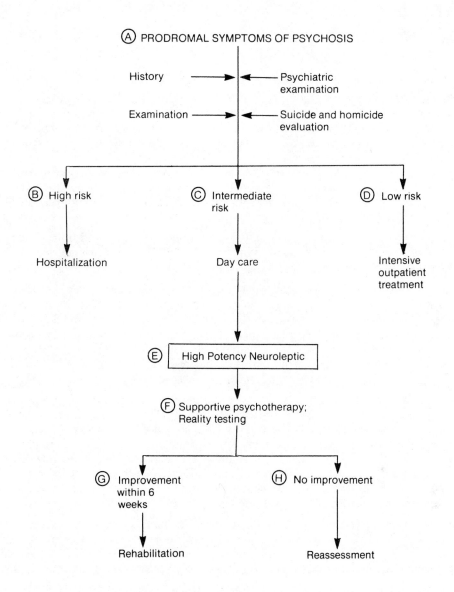

(A) PRODROMAL SYMPTOMS OF PSYCHOSIS

History ——→ ←—— Psychiatric examination

Examination ——→ ←—— Suicide and homicide evaluation

(B) High risk   (C) Intermediate risk   (D) Low risk

Hospitalization   Day care   Intensive outpatient treatment

(E) High Potency Neuroleptic

(F) Supportive psychotherapy; Reality testing

(G) Improvement within 6 weeks   (H) No improvement

Rehabilitation   Reassessment

with medication should be monitored by obtaining blood levels. Hospitalization, changing medication, prescribing higher doses, behavior therapy to reward better functioning, and in some cases, ECT, should be considered in agitated and suicidal schizophrenic patients who do not improve.

REFERENCES

Groves JE. Psychotic and borderline patients. In: Cassem Hackett, eds. Handbook of General Hospital Psychiatry. St. Louis: CV Mosby, 1978: 174.
Croughan JL, Woodruff RA, Reich T. The management of patients with undiagnosed psychiatric illness. Arch Gen Psychiatry, 1979; 36:341.

MANIA

Deborah A. Coyle, M.D.

COMMENTS

A. Manic episodes may occur spontaneously or may be precipitated by antidepressants in patients with a past history of mania. They tend to last 3–6 months without treatment. Mania is characterized by a distinct period of predominantly elevated, expansive, or irritable mood lasting at least one week and accompanied by at least 3 of the following symptoms: increased activity or physical restlessness, rapid, pressured speech, flight of ideas, inflated self-esteem, decreased need for sleep, distractability, and involvement in activities that have a high potential for painful consequences. Hypomania is a pathologic disturbance less severe than mania. Ongoing evaluation of dangerousness (pp 20–21) is necessary to protect patient and staff.

B. Differentiation of mania from other agitated psychoses is summarized on p 29. Physical conditions that may produce manic symptoms include hemodialysisenelzine, digitalis, cocaine, and amphetamines.

C. Manic patients who exhibit loss of reality testing, delusions, hallucinations, poor judgment, or unpredictable or dangerous behavior require hospitalization. If lack of insight, overestimation of their strengths and enjoyment of elated mood lead the patient to refuse hospitalization and treatment, involuntary treatment should be arranged. Initial hospital care involves reduction of environmental stressors, lithium carbonate (1200–2400 mg/day to achieve a blood level of 0.8–1.2 mEq/L), neuroleptics to control agitation until lithium begins to take effect (often 7–10 days), and restraint (pp 14–15) when necessary.

D. Failure to respond to lithium may indicate another psychosis, especially schizophrenia or organic brain syndrome (organic affective syndrome). The 30% of manics who do not respond to lithium can usually be treated with high doses of antipsychotics. In life-threatening mania, electroconvulsive therapy is dramatically effective. Carbamazepine, clonidine, propranolol, and calcium antagonists are investigational antimanic drugs for refractory mania. Outpatient management should only be attempted if the patient will comply with medications, if patient symptoms are mild (i.e., hypomania), and if reliable family members and friends work with the therapist.

E. Hypomanic patients have fair judgment and experience manic symptoms not severe enough to warrant hospitalization. If a reliable family member or friend is available and the patient appears for regular appointments, lithium carbonate and psychotherapy may be administered on an outpatient basis with close observation for signs of deterioration.

F. Maintenance lithium therapy is 600–1800 mg/day to achieve a blood level of 0.5–1.0 mEq/L 12 hours after dosage and should be continued for 1 year. To prolong lithium therapy beyond 1 year, the therapist must weigh the medical risks (particularly renal) versus the hazards of manic relapse (particularly violence and psychosocial sequelae such as termination from work, divorce). Tricyclics, alcohol, and street drugs increase the risk of manic relapse. Patients should be seen monthly. During the visit, obtain careful interval medical history, looking specifically for CNS, renal, hypothyroid, cardiac, and dermatological complications of lithium therapy. Laboratory checks should include monthly lithium serum level (at 12 hours after last dose), urinalysis, urine volume, serum electrolytes, serum creatinine, T4, and TSH. Change in sodium intake, fluid intake, or concomitant use of medications (particularly diuretics) can dramatically alter serum lithium level. Since patients frequently discontinue lithium prematurely, several lithium checks should be random and unannounced. Outpatient psychotherapy helps the patient identify precipitants and early symptoms of mania. Sensitivity to loss and fragile self-esteem also must be frequently addressed. Families should be educated regarding prodromal signs of mania and allowed to discuss the disruptive effects on the family. Manic patients can be quite impaired in their abilities as spouse and parent.

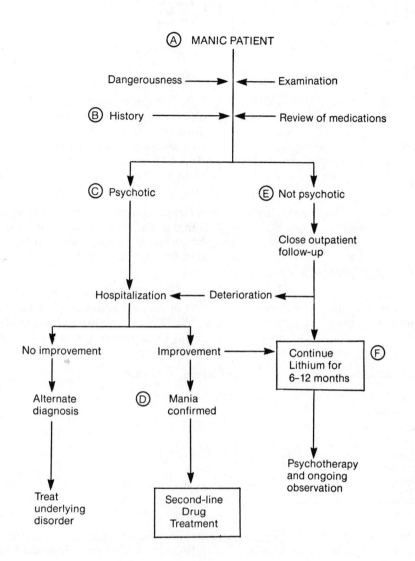

(A) MANIC PATIENT

Dangerousness ⟶ ⟵ Examination

(B) History ⟶ ⟵ Review of medications

(C) Psychotic

(E) Not psychotic

Close outpatient follow-up

Hospitalization ⟵ Deterioration ⟵

No improvement

Improvement ⟶

(F) Continue Lithium for 6–12 months

Alternate diagnosis

(D) Mania confirmed

Treat underlying disorder

Second-line Drug Treatment

Psychotherapy and ongoing observation

REFERENCES

Carlson GA, Goodwin FK. The stages of mania. Arch Gen Psychiatry 1973; 28:221–225.
Klerman GL. Overview of affective disorders. In: Kaplan HI, Freedman Am, Sadock BJ, eds. Comprehensive Textbook of Psychiatry. 3rd ed. Baltimore: Williams & Wilkins, 1980: 1305–1330.
Krauthammer C, Klerman GL. Secondary mania. Arch Gen Psychiatry 1978; 35:1333–1337.
Wing J, Mixon J. Discriminating symptoms in schizophrenia. Arch Gen Psychiatry 1975; 32:853–857.

LITHIUM CARBONATE

Steven L. Dubovsky, M.D.

COMMENTS

Lithium carbonate is effective in about 70 percent of acutely manic patients. It also may prevent recurrent manic attacks, as well as recurrent depression in patients with bipolar disorder. Its usefulness in the treatment of acute depression is more controversial. Because lithium causes neutrophilia it is sometimes used to treat neutropenia associated with cancer chemotherapy. Lithium has a role in the prophylaxis of cluster headache. Its antagonism of the renal action of vasopressin makes it effective in ameliorating the syndrome of inappropriate secretion of anti-diuretic hormone.

Any diuretic that causes loss of sodium will result in increased renal conservation of lithium as well as sodium, resulting in increased blood levels of lithium. The same phenomenon is produced by excess sweating or other causes of sodium loss. Patients taking lithium should avoid low salt diets. Lithium levels are also increased by tetracycline, indomethacin, and methyldopa; blood levels are decreased by phenothiazines.

Reports of a variety of irreversible neurologic syndromes in patients taking lithium and haloperidol mandate caution and careful observation of patients taking this combination. A significant number of patients taking antidepressants plus lithium develop rapid cycling of mania and depression; limiting the long-term usefulness of this combination. It is unknown whether newer antimanic drugs combined with antidepressants will produce the same effect.

In therapeutic doses, lithium may produce the following side effects:

> Nausea, vomiting, diarrhea, abdominal pain
> A dazed, tired feeling
> Fine tremor
> Thirst, polyuria
> Nephrogenic diabetes insipidus
> Nontoxic goiter
> Weight gain
> Hyperparathyroidism
> Leukocytosis

Although the issue is controversial, lithium does seem to have the potential to produce irreversible renal tubular damage of uncertain significance. Utilizing the lowest possible blood level and obtaining periodic measures of urine volume and serum creatinine therefore seem prudent. Lithium is teratogenic, its most devastating effort being on the cardiovascular system (Ebstein's anomaly). It is excreted in breast milk; its effects on the newborn are unknown. Lithium can prolong the action of succinylcholine.

Lithium toxicity, which usually occurs at blood levels > 2 mEq/l but may be seen at lower blood levels, is associated with: decreased muscle tone, fasciculations, delirium, and coma.

Osmotic diuresis to speed excretion, administration of large amounts of sodium, or dialysis, may be used to clear excess lithium if the patient's life is in danger.

REFERENCES

Klein DF, Gittelman R, Quitkin F, Rifkin A. Diagnosis and Drug Treatment of Psychiatric Disorders: Adults and Children. 2nd ed. Baltimore: Williams & Wilkins, 1982.
Baldessarini RJ. Drugs and the treatment of psychiatric disorders. In: Gilman AG, Goodman LS, Gilman A, eds. The Pharmacological Basis of Therapeutics. New York: Macmillan, 1980: 391–447.

LITHIUM CARBONATE

Usual Daily Dose

900-2400 mg

Serum concentration =
0.5–1.2 mEq/1 for
accute mania;
0.4–0.8 mEq/1 for
prophylaxis

*Special Characteristics
and Indications*

Proven effective
for management and
prophylaxis of mania

Useful in prevention of
recurrent depression with
past history of mania (bipolar
depression) and some recurrent
unipolar depressions

May by useful in
treatment of some
acute depressions

Useful for management
of cluster headache,
neutropenia, and syndrome
of inappropriate ADH secretion

CHRONIC DEPRESSION

Jeffrey L. Metzner, M.D.

COMMENTS

A. Chronic depression is a dysphoric mood lasting at least 6 months associated with loss of interest or pleasure in usual activities, guilt, lowered self-esteem, hopelessness, helplessness, vegetative signs, and suicidal thoughts. Major affective disorder (primary depression) is not associated with any other medical, surgical, or psychiatric illness. Syndromes of depression include major depressive disorder, bipolar disorder (depression with a past history of mania), cyclothymic disorder (at least a 2-year history of recurrent episodes of depression and hypomania but less severe than bipolar disorder or major depression), dysthymic disorder (at least 2-year history of depressive symptoms not severe enough to meet criteria for major depression), and atypical affective disorder (affective symptoms that do not meet criteria for other disorders). Secondary depression occurs in the context of another illness or disorder, especially thyroid, adrenal, and pituitary disease, viral infections, tumors, metabolic disturbances, dementia, chronic pain, and schizophrenia. Drugs that may cause depression include antihypertensives, CNS depressants, adrenal steroids, oral contraceptives, and alcohol; withdrawal from CNS stimulants also may cause depression (pp 56–57).

B. Dynamic psychotherapy is indicated to attempt to resolve emotional conflicts that result in continued depression. Important issues may include guilt, helplessness, passivity, negative expectations, dependency, anger, and disappointment. Some patients benefit from a behavioral approach in which depressive behaviors are ignored by therapist and family while nondepressive behaviors are rewarded. Cognitive therapy, in which the patient is confronted with the unrealistic nature of his negative perceptions, may also be helpful. Somatic therapy of depression is discussed on pages 58 through 62.

C. If aggressive psychiatric treatment or medical/surgical therapy is ineffective, symptoms may be due to a different psychiatric disorder. This possibility is enhanced by the presence of feelings of emptiness, meaninglessness, unrealistic idealization, devaluation, intense anger, delusions, and hallucinations.

D. Depression is frequently described by patients with borderline, narcissistic, passive aggressive, and antisocial personality disorders. Careful questioning usually reveals feelings of emptiness with which it is difficult to empathize rather than the sadness of primary depression. Problems in interpersonal relationships, including the doctor-patient relationship, frequently precipitate complaints of depression in patients with personality disorders. Drugs that may be habituating or that may worsen depression must be avoided. Psychotherapy should focus on real-life problems rather than the patient's fantasies, and the therapist should be consistently available. It may be impossible to resolve suffering that provides a focus for the patient's life, regular contact with others, and serves other important psychological functions.

E. Somatization disorder (recurrent and varied complaints in multiple systems), hypochondriasis (preoccupation with the fear or belief of having a serious physical disorder), and psychogenic pain disorder (persistent nonorganic pain) are commonly accompanied by unhappiness and emptiness. These symptoms are related to unmet dependency needs, loneliness, and emotional deprivation. The patient should be assured of an ongoing relationship with a physician who acknowledges that the patient is ill (pp 84–85).

REFERENCES

Dubovsky SL, Weissberg MP. Clinical Psychiatry in Primary Care. 2nd ed. Baltimore: Williams & Wilkins, 1982.
Dubovsky SL. Psychotherapeutics in Primary Care. New York: Grune & Stratton, 1981.
Krupp NE. Psychiatric Aspects of Chronic and Crippling Illness. Psychosomatics 1968; 9:109–113.

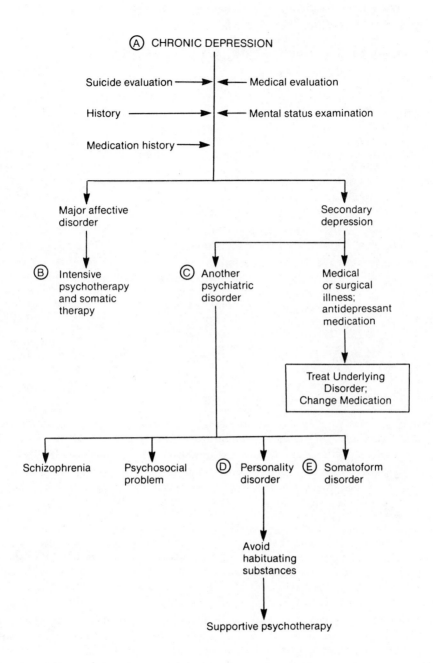

(A) CHRONIC DEPRESSION

Suicide evaluation ⟶ ⟵ Medical evaluation

History ⟶ ⟵ Mental status examination

Medication history ⟶

Major affective disorder

Secondary depression

(B) Intensive psychotherapy and somatic therapy

(C) Another psychiatric disorder

Medical or surgical illness; antidepressant medication

Treat Underlying Disorder; Change Medication

Schizophrenia

Psychosocial problem

(D) Personality disorder

(E) Somatoform disorder

Avoid habituating substances

Supportive psychotherapy

CHRONIC SEVERE SELF-DESTRUCTIVE BEHAVIOR

Steven L. Dubovsky, M.D.

COMMENTS

A. In contrast with more subtle forms of self-destructive behavior such as smoking and overeating, chronic suicide attempts, nonsuicidal forms of self-mutilation (e.g., wrist cutting), and purposeful worsening of dangerous illnesses command the physician's immediate attention. Past and family history of psychiatric disorder may reveal inadequately treated acute depression, delirium, or psychosis. Self-destructive behavior also may be an attempt to control chronic psychotic thoughts or intolerable emotions. Impulsivity caused by a chronic organic brain syndrome may lead to self-destructive acts. Alcohol and sedating drugs decrease impulse control and make dangerous behavior more likely.

B. Family members may covertly encourage self-destructive behavior. Hopelessness, unrealistic therapeutic goals, and anger interfere with the physician's ability to diagnose the problem dispassionately and accept the limitations of current treatment techniques.

C. Serious exacerbations of habitual self-destructive patterns and emergence of behaviors not in the patient's usual repertoire indicate worsening of the patient's condition or a new illness that requires his protection and intensive treatment. Although they are not cured, most patients are able to return to an unstable baseline. If life-threatening behavior continues after the crisis has resolved or intercurrent depression or acute psychosis has been vigorously treated, long-term custodial care may be necessary. Rapid stabilization may occur when the patient realizes he will not receive acute attention indefinitely.

D. While acute suicidal behavior requires immediate intervention, responding rapidly to long-standing self-destructive behavior may encourage the patient to communicate with behavior that captures the physician's attention rather than with words, which are less dramatic.

E. Self-injurious behavior may be a response to command hallucinations, a search for delusional infestations, an attempt to relieve feelings of unreality, a means of distraction from psychological pain, or an expression of hopelessness in chronic schizophrenic or psychotically depressed patients.

F. The chronically self-destructive patient with borderline or related personality disorder uses self-destructive behavior to relieve inner tension, control others, and communicate distress. If the patient has not been receiving regular psychiatric treatment, ongoing psychotherapy may help to decrease self-destructive behavior. Confrontation is essential to successful treatment.

G. The patient who becomes more self-destructive while in psychotherapy may use self-destructive behavior to keep the therapist's attention or to signal his discomfort with the intensity of the therapeutic interaction. The therapist should avoid rewarding the behavior with more frequent appointments or other forms of increased attention. At the same time, he should convey an interest in whatever feelings the patient might wish to convey in words rather than actions. Since self-destructive behavior that develops or worsens during psychotherapy is often a reaction to feelings about intimacy provoked by the doctor-patient relationship, discussion should focus on the patient's wish to control, express anger with, or escape from, the physician. If behavior continues, the intensity of treatment should be decreased, at least temporarily, through less frequent visits or a trial of no psychiatric treatment. If self-destructive symptoms develop in the context of ongoing medical therapy, any necessary treatment should be provided by another physician or clinic.

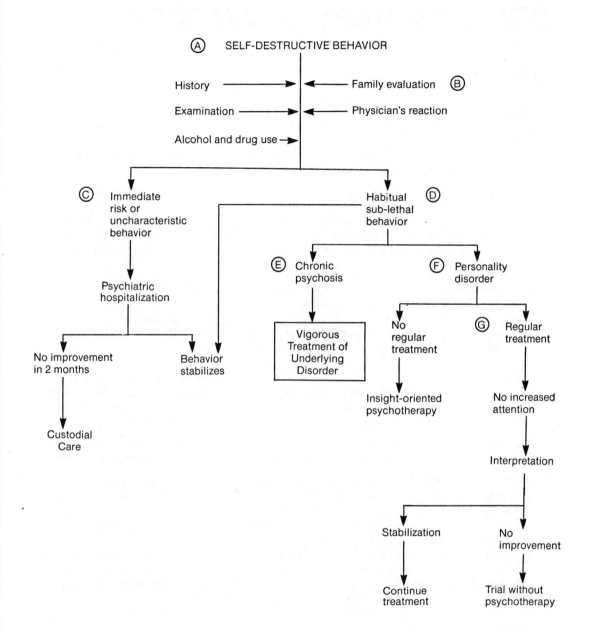

(A) SELF-DESTRUCTIVE BEHAVIOR

History ⟶ ⟵ Family evaluation (B)

Examination ⟶ ⟵ Physician's reaction

Alcohol and drug use ⟶

(C) Immediate risk or uncharacteristic behavior

(D) Habitual sub-lethal behavior

Psychiatric hospitalization

(E) Chronic psychosis

(F) Personality disorder

No improvement in 2 months

Behavior stabilizes

Vigorous Treatment of Underlying Disorder

No regular treatment

(G) Regular treatment

Custodial Care

Insight-oriented psychotherapy

No increased attention

Interpretation

Stabilization

No improvement

Continue treatment

Trial without psychotherapy

REFERENCES

Abt LE, Weissman SL. Acting Out. New York: Grune & Stratton, 1965.

Schwartz DA, Flinn DE, Slawson PF. Treatment of the suicidal character. Amer J Psychother 1974; 28:195–207.

Kernberg OF. Borderline Conditions and Pathological Narcissism. New York: Jason Aronson, 1975.

DRUG THERAPY OF ANXIETY
Alan Feiger, M.D.

COMMENTS

A. Having excluded medical and psychiatric illnesses and medications that may produce anxiety (pp 52–53), it is important to determine whether anxiety is exogenous (evoked by some precipitating stress or psychological conflict) or endogenous (occurs spontaneously). Panic attacks and some phobias are endogenous in that they do not arise in response to an obvious external or internal psychological stressor (pp 52–53).

B. In usual antidepressant doses, imipramine, desipramine, maprotiline, and trazodone may abort panic attacks within 1 month. Alprazolam is a new triazobenzodiazepine that appears to ameliorate some panic attacks and depression. Although probably no more effective than tricyclics or MAO inhibitors, alprazolam is safe, well tolerated, and should produce improvement within 2 weeks. It must be withdrawn very slowly to avoid withdrawal seizures.

C. MAO inhibitors (pp 64–65) are more reliable than other medications in relieving panic attacks and other forms of endogenous anxiety. However, because strict dietary precautions must be observed, these drugs are usually prescribed only if standard antidepressants or alprazolam have not been effective. Patients who amplify the physical sensations that normally accompany anxiety, for example, paresthesias and faintness, may be more likely to respond to an MAO inhibitor, even if anxiety seems exogenous.

D. Failure to improve substantially indicates that the diagnosis and/or the treatment are incorrect and further investigation is necessary. If improvement is complete, medications should be withdrawn gradually after 6 months. If symptoms return, the original dosage should be reinstituted for another 3 to 6 months and drug withdrawal attempted again.

E. Patients with a delayed, prolonged response to a stress that would make most people anxious (post-traumatic stress disorder) respond better to MAO inhibitors than to benzodiazepines.

F. Benzodiazepines (pp 68–69) are most effective when they are prescribed for less than 1 month to a patient with a clearcut psychosocial stress that is likely to abate. However, patients with limited ability to resolve conflicts or those under prolonged stress may need maintenance treatment. The risk of creating addiction is low in these circumstances. Long-acting preparations such as diazepam and chlordiazepoxide produce less rebound anxiety than do slower-acting preparations. Drug withdrawal is also easier, although abstinence syndromes may appear 10 to 14 days after discontinuation of the drug. Oxazepam, lorazepam, and other compounds with shorter half-lives are less likely than longer-acting drugs to result in oversedation or drug accumulation in patients with impaired hepatic or cerebral function and patients using drugs such as cimetidine or oral contraceptives that increase the blood levels of longer-acting preparations.

G. The sedative side effects of antihistamines decrease anxiety less predictably than do benzodiazepines, but the risk of addiction in patients with a history of drug or alcohol abuse or with antisocial personality is minimal.

H. Stage fright and anxiety associated with marked tremor and tachycardia may be reduced with a beta-blocking agent such as propranolol, although anxiety reduction is less predictable than with benzodiazepines.

REFERENCES

Sheehan DV. Current perspectives in the treatment of panic and phobic disorders. Drug Ther 1982; :49.
Klein DF, Gittelman R, Quitkin F, Rifkin A.
Diagnosis and Drug Treatment of Psychiatric Disorders: Adults and Children.
Baltimore: Williams & Wilkins, 1980: 493.

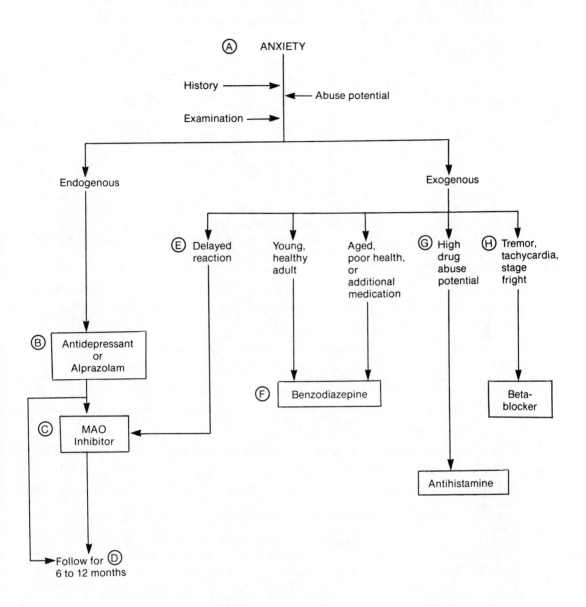

ANXIETY

(A)

History ———→

←——— Abuse potential

Examination ———→

Endogenous

Exogenous

(E) Delayed reaction

Young, healthy adult

Aged, poor health, or additional medication

(G) High drug abuse potential

(H) Tremor, tachycardia, stage fright

(B) Antidepressant or Alprazolam

(F) Benzodiazepine

Beta-blocker

(C) MAO Inhibitor

Antihistamine

Follow for (D) 6 to 12 months

Marks I. Fears and Phobias. New York: Academic Press, 1969.
Bernstein JG. Antianxiety agents and hypnotics. In: Handbook of Drug Therapy in Psychiatry. Littleton, MA: John Wright, 1983: 23.

GENERAL APPROACH TO ANXIETY

Alan Feiger, M.D.

COMMENTS

A. Anxiety is a sense of subjective dread tht may be accompanied by signs of autonomic arousal and that is out of proportion to any precipitating situation. The use of antianxiety medications as a primary or adjunctive modality is summarized on pp 50–51. Common (9–40%) medical causes include side effects of drugs (caffeine, theophylline, amphetamine, cocaine, hallucinogens, PCP, and motor restlessness caused by antipsychotic drugs); withdrawal from alcohol, benzodiazepines, sedative hypnotics, and antidepressants; cardiovascular conditions; endocrinopathies; neurologic disorders; and respiratory conditions. Psychiatric disorders frequently associated with prominent anxiety include depression, schizophrenia, mania, and somatoform disorders such as hypochondriasis.

B. Endogenous anxiety arises spontaneously rather than in response to an external stress. Panic attacks, the principle form of endogenous anxiety, are spontaneous episodes of severe apprehension accompanied by at least 4 of the following symptoms: dyspnea, palpitations, chest pain, sensation of choking or smothering, dizziness, vertigo or unsteadiness, feelings of unreality, paresthesias, sensations of hot or cold, sweating, fainting, trembling, and fear of dying or losing one's mind. Diagnosis may be facilitated by the appearance of symptoms such as hyperventilation or lactate infusion. After repeated panic attacks, patients may develop anticipatory anxiety, phobic avoidance of potential anxiety-provoking situations, depression due to lack of improvement, hypochondriasis, dependency on the physician, and compulsive rituals in an attempt to control anxiety. Phobias may also have an endogenous quality if they are not symbolic of an unconscious conflict and do not develop after a frightening experience. Endogenous forms of anxiety tend to respond best to tricyclic and related antidepressants, alprazolam, and MAO inhibitors (pp 64–65).

C. Substance abuse may develop as the patient attempts unsuccessfully to control anxiety with sedatives or alcohol. A period of abstinence is necessary to distinguish withdrawal symptoms associated with drug discontinuation from a return of preexisting anxiety.

D. Phobias of specific situations are treated by controlled exposure to the frightening situation, first in fantasy and then in reality. In systematic desensitization, the patient pairs relaxation, usually induced by hypnosis, with imagining progressively more anxiety-provoking situations until he can picture himself in the upsetting environment without feeling anxious. Gradual exposure to the actual situation with the therapist or other supportive figure present is then added.

E. Exogenous anxiety is a response to a psychosocial stress, although malingering for financial compensation or drugs should be considered. An apparently minor event may have important symbolic meaning that triggers unresolved emotional conflicts and precipitates anxiety. Reactions to severe stresses may be immediate (adjustment disorder), or they may be delayed 3 months or more (post-traumatic stress disorder). Insight-oriented psychotherapy helps identify the unconscious meaning of the situation. Psychological support, relaxation training, biofeedback, advice about avoiding anxiety-provoking situations, and environment manipulation are necessary when the patient cannot or does not wish to resolve conflicts. For post-traumatic stress disorders refractory to psychological intervention, tricyclics and MAO inhibitors are useful.

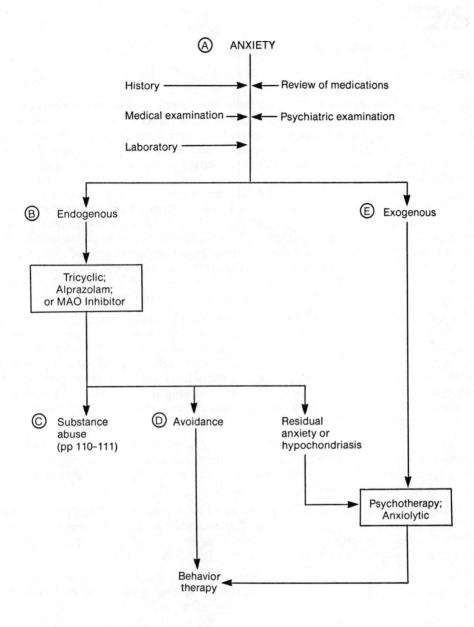

REFERENCE

Marks I. Fears and Phobias. New York: Academic Press, 1969.

GRIEF

Janice Petersen, M.D.

COMMENTS

A. Grief is a normal reaction to loss of a loved one, health, status, employment, financial security, or an ideal. Symptoms include sadness, crying, preoccupation with the lost person, anger, anxiety, social withdrawal, feelings that the patient should have been able to do more for the lost person or should not have survived, and difficulty in sleeping, eating and working. Physical symptoms mimicking those of the deceased are not uncommon, and vivid dreams or even hallucinations of the deceased may occur. Grief is usually acute for 4 to 6 weeks, gradually decreasing in intensity over the following year but returning at anniversaries of the loss. Sometimes, symptoms appear for the first time at an anniversary or other symbolic date. Previous unresolved losses, conflicts with the person who has died, and latent psychiatric problems can result in complicated grief reactions. Morbidity and mortality from medical illnesses are higher in the bereaved than in the general population; elective surgical procedures should be deferred during acute grief in order to minimize complications. Since the suicide rate is increased in bereaved patients (often out of a wish to join the lost person), evaluation of suicide potential is essential in the assessment of the grieving patient.

B. The patient should be encouraged to allow mourning to run its course in order to avoid depression, chronic physical complaints, and other complications of unexpressed grief. He should be reassured that even though the experience is painful, he will feel better if he permits himself to continue grieving. Grieving is facilitated by talking about the lost person and expressing the emotions the patient is experiencing. Hypnotics may be prescribed for insomnia, but daytime sedation interferes with mourning and should be avoided. Support groups may be helpful to patients who feel isolated or who are afraid that they will not be able to tolerate grief.

C. Patients may avoid grief because it feels too painful, it threatens to evoke severe psychiatric symptoms or because personality deficits make them incapable of experiencing normal grief. Active discussions of feelings, about the deceased, and of the reasons why the patient is afraid of mourning, may help to precipitate active grief.

D. Like any severe stress, bereavement may precipitate or exacerbate latent psychiatric disorders such as psychoses or personality disorders that undermine the patient's ability to cope with stress. Aggressive treatment of the underlying disorder is necessary to help to organize the patient psychologically so that he may proceed with normal grieving.

E. When marked sadness or withdrawal persist for more than 6 months, or hopelessness, apathy, hyperactivity, generalized anger and self-punitive behavior become evident, grief has become excessive. Antidepressants (pp 62–63) should be considered if early morning awakening, unrealistic guilt, lowered self-esteem, and past history or family history of depression are present or if symptoms persist despite adequate psychotherapy.

REFERENCES

Greenblatt M. The grieving spouse. Amer J Psychiatry 1978; 135:43–47.
Wittkower E, Warnes H, eds. Psychosomatic Medicine. New York: Harper & Row, 1977.

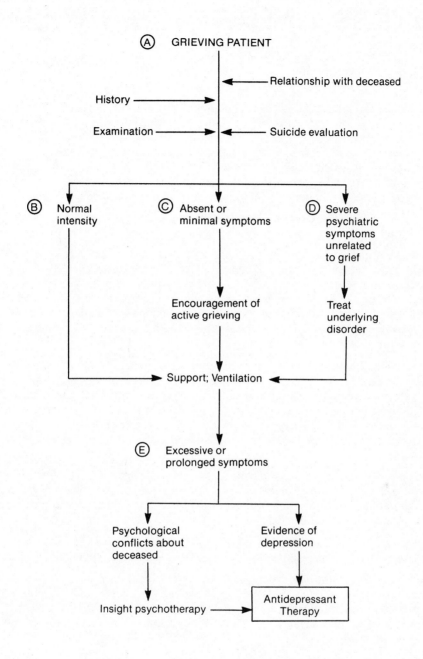

A GRIEVING PATIENT

Relationship with deceased

History

Examination ← Suicide evaluation

B Normal intensity

C Absent or minimal symptoms

D Severe psychiatric symptoms unrelated to grief

Encouragement of active grieving

Treat underlying disorder

Support; Ventilation

E Excessive or prolonged symptoms

Psychological conflicts about deceased

Evidence of depression

Insight psychotherapy → Antidepressant Therapy

SADNESS, UNHAPPINESS, MISERY

Steven L. Dubovsky, M.D.

COMMENTS

A. Recent losses, past history, family history of depression, and chronicity of symptoms help to distinguish depression from other entities. Illnesses in which depression may be a presenting complaint include: hyper- or hydroadrenalism, hypercalcemia, pernicious anemia, pancreatic carcinoma, viral infections, systemic lupus erythematosus, hypothyroidism, and organic brain syndrome of any cause. Drugs that can cause depression include: adrenal steroids and ACTH, antihypertensives (e.g., reserpine, methyldopa, spironolactone), L-dopa, propranolol, barbiturates and minor tranquilizers, oral contraceptives, and alcohol.

B. Suicide potential *must* be evaluated in *all* patients who are upset, unhappy, or depressed.

C. Grief is a normal reaction to the loss of a valued person, object, ideal, or status. It is characterized by sadness, painful preoccupation with the lost person that comes and goes in waves, insomnia, restlessness, somatic distress, and anger, often at the physician. Normal grief is acute for 4–6 weeks; some symptoms may persist up to a year, with recurrence at important anniversaries. Grief is facilitated by encouraging the patient to talk about the loss. A benzodiazepine hypnotic is appropriate, but daytime sedation and other attempts to suppress mourning should be avoided.

D. Depression is differentiated from grief by the presence of guilt, lowered self-esteem, hopelessness, helplessness, anger turned against the self, and vegetative signs. Depression may complicate grief when the relationship with the lost person was ambivalent, when the loss occurred under unusual circumstances (e.g., by suicide), or when the patient is biologically predisposed. Psychotherapy helps the patient to become aware of dependency wishes, anger turned against the self, passivity, self punishment, and a desire to feel better without having to work at it.

E. Predictors of possible response to an antidepressant include: past history or family history of response to somatic therapy, family history of affective disorder, prominent vegetative signs, severe symptoms, positive dexamethasone suppression test, and expectation of the patient that an antidepressant will be effective.

F. Symptoms may recur if treatment is discontinued too early. As many as 40 to 90 percent of acutely depressed patients who recover completely have been said to relapse within 2 years.

G. In addition to developing depression when they appreciate the seriousness of their illnesses, patients with schizophrenia and those with some personality disorders may express dysphoria that is distinguished from true depression by emptiness and an inability to communicate true depth of emotion to the examiner. Organic brain syndromes may mimic primary depression.

H. As many as 40 percent of depressions may become chronic despite adequate treatment. Although they may improve initially with any treatment, patients who are continuously depressed for years because they need chronic physical and/or mental impairment and suffering to organize their lives, excuse their failures, ensure caretaking, and provide ongoing punishment may resist attempts to remove their symptoms, resulting in an inevitable return of distress. Treatment is similar to the approach to the hypochondriacal patient.

REFERENCES

Friedman RJ, Katz M, eds. Depression and Human Existence. Boston: Little, Brown, 1975.
Plath S. The Bell Jar. New York: Harper & Row, 1971.

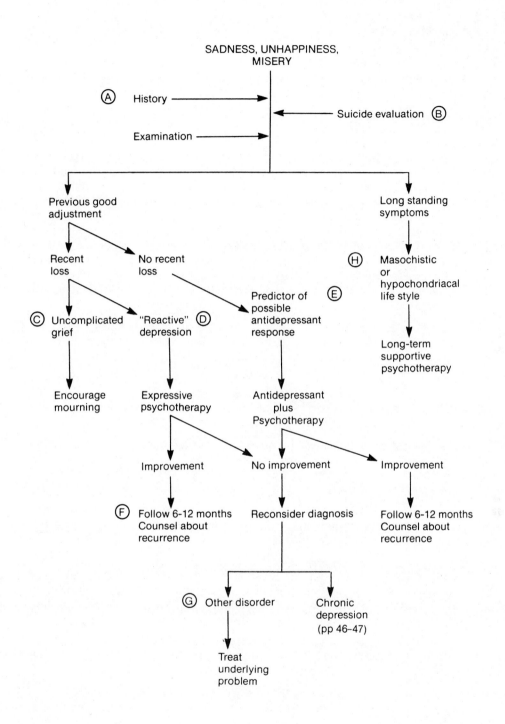

SADNESS, UNHAPPINESS,
MISERY

(A) History

Examination

Suicide evaluation (B)

Previous good
adjustment

Long standing
symptoms

Recent
loss

No recent
loss

(H) Masochistic
or
hypochondriacal
life style

(E)
Predictor of
possible
antidepressant
response

(C) Uncomplicated
grief

"Reactive" (D)
depression

Long-term
supportive
psychotherapy

Encourage
mourning

Expressive
psychotherapy

Antidepressant
plus
Psychotherapy

Improvement

No improvement

Improvement

(F) Follow 6-12 months
Counsel about
recurrence

Reconsider diagnosis

Follow 6-12 months
Counsel about
recurrence

(G) Other disorder

Chronic
depression
(pp 46–47)

Treat
underlying
problem

Rush J, ed. Short-term Psychotherapies for Depression. Boston: Guilford Press, 1982.
Klerman GJ. Overview of affective disorders. In: Kaplan HI, Freedman AM, Sadock BJ, eds.
    Comprehensive Textbook of Psychiatry. 3rd ed. Baltimore: Williams & Wilkins, 1980: 1305–1319.

SOMATIC THERAPY OF DEPRESSION

Alan Feiger, M.D.

COMMENTS

A. The depressed patient with indications for somatic therapy (pp 56, 60) should be given an antidepressant to which the patient or a family member has responded in the past. However, a history of a poor response to a particular drug may reflect inadequate dosage rather than the incorrect medication. In the absence of suggestive factors from the history, antidepressants are chosen according to their side effects and the physician's familiarity with them. Depressed patients with associated anxiety or insomnia should receive a sedating antidepressant such as amitriptyline or trazodone; retarded depressions may respond to more activating drugs such as protriptyline or maprotiline. Trazodone, desipramine, and maprotiline are least anticholinergic. Some clinicians feel that patients with low 24-hour urinary excretion of 3-methoxy- 4-hydroxyl-phenylglycol (MHPG), a metabolite of norepinephrine, and patients with transient mood elevation in response to amphetamines, are more likely to respond to a nonadrenergic antidepressant such as desipramine, doxepin, or maprotiline.

B. ECT should be considered as the initial treatment if the patient is imminently suicidal, severely depressed, unable to tolerate the cardiovascular side effects of antidepressants, over age 70, or has a past history of response to ECT but not to antidepressants.

C. In the absence of other indications, psychomotor retardation is the best indicator of potential response to an antidepressant. Early morning awakening, diurnal mood swing, loss of reactivity to the environment, and persistent anhedonia are additional predictors of response to an antidepressant.

D. Patients with a past history of mania may become manic if they are treated with antidepressants alone. However, rapid cycling (frequently alternating depression and mania) may develop when lithium and antidepressants are prescribed together for prolonged periods of time.

E. Depression associated with hyperphagia, weight gain, hypersomnia, self-pity, phobias, sensitivity to rejection, and somatic symptoms of anxiety responds best to MAO inhibitors, but 50% of patients may show no improvement.

F. Healthy patients should be started on a tricyclic or related drug by prescribing 50 mg of amitriptyline or its equivalent, taken at bedtime. The dose should be increased by 50 mg every 3 days to a maximum dose of 300 mg of amitriptyline per day or its equivalent, until depression improves or until side effects preclude further treatment.

G. Failure to respond to initial somatic therapy is discussed on pp 60–61. Organic brain syndromes, hostile families, personality disorders, and subtle hypothyroidism are additional causes of treatment-resistant depression.

H. Unilateral (nondominant) ECT produces less memory loss but is not always as effective as bilateral ECT. Continuing drug therapy following a course of ECT reduces the relapse rate by 20-50%. Two months after ECT, the dose of antidepressant should be decreased by 10% per week until it is 50% of the initial level or until depressive symptoms reemerge. The drug should be discontinued after 6-8 months unless the patient has a history of frequent, severe depressions or an abnormal DST does not return to normal.

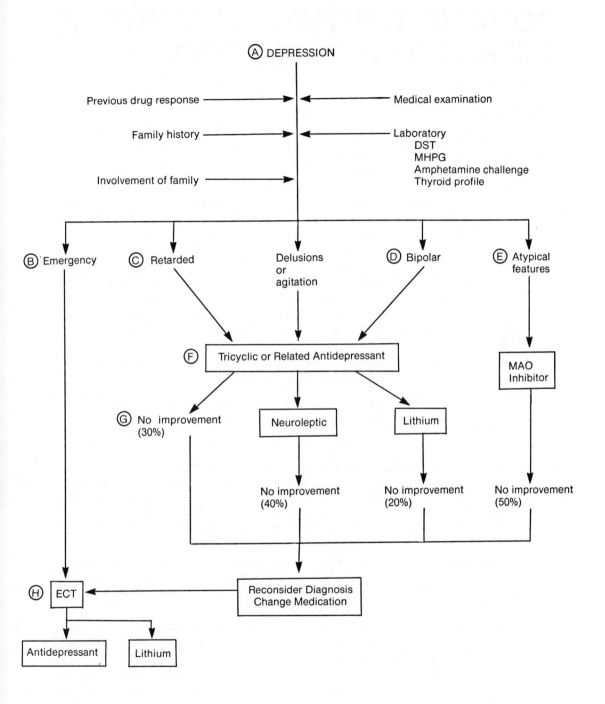

REFERENCES

Bernstein J. Handbook of Drug Therapy in Psychiatry. New York: John Wright Publishers, 1983.
Ayd F. Affective Disorders Reassessed. Baltimore: Ayd Publications, 1983.
Greenspoon L, ed. Psychiatry Update. Washington DC: American Psychiatric Press, 1983.

SOMATIC THERAPY OF TRICYCLIC REFRACTORY DEPRESSION

Alan Feiger, M.D.

COMMENTS

A. Thirty percent of depressed patients do not respond to appropriately administered tricyclic antidepressants. Inadequate dosage, noncompliance and misdiagnosis are the most common causes of resistance to antidepressants. Old age, chronic symptoms, delusions, anxiety, concurrent panic attacks, and alcoholism increase the likelihood of resistance to tricyclics. A past history or family history of failure to respond to a particular antidepressant suggests that the patient will not benefit from that drug. Depression produced by medications and physical illnesses (pp 56–57) may not respond to antidepressants.

B. The emotional withdrawal, apathy, confusion, and emptiness associated with schizophrenia, dementia, or borderline personality may mimic primary depression but are less likely to respond to antidepressants than are more clear-cut depressive syndromes. However, when vegetative signs, guilt, and lowered self-esteem are prominent, secondary depression in these patients may respond to the appropriate antidepressant. An adequate tricyclic trial is 5 weeks of a minimum of 150 mg daily of imipramine or its equivalent.
equivalent.

C. Blood levels are useful in determining compliance and in assessing appropriate dosages of nortriptyline, amitriptyline, imipramine, and possibly desipramine.

D. Some authorities recommend changing from a serotonergic (amitriptyline, trazodone) to a noradrenergic (imipramine, maprotiline) antidepressant or vice-versa. Others recommend proceeding immediately to an MAO inhibitor, a newer antidepressant (alprazolam or bupropion) or, in severe cases, electroconvulsive therapy (ECT).

E. MAO inhibitors are particularly likely to be effective when depressive symptoms are associated with increased appetite, weight gain, hypersomnia, hypochondriacal symptoms, panic attacks, and chronic pain. Lithium or small doses (25 μg) of T_3 may be added to tricyclics or MAO inhibitors. Short-term administration of methylphenidate or amphetamine-which cannot be combined with any antidepressants-produces improvement in some depressed, physically ill patients.

F. Patients with delusional or agitated depressions have a better initial response to antipsychotic drugs, especially chlorpromazine, thioridazine, thiothixene and loxapine, with or without tricyclics, than to tricyclics alone. The neuroleptic should be discontinued when delusions and agitations abate, in order to prevent tardive dyskinesia.

G. Seventy percent of depressed patients who do not improve with medication respond to ECT. ECT should be the initial treatment for depression with severe suicide risk, rapidly deteriorating course, medical complications, or profound withdrawal. It should be considered early in patients with a past history or family history of response to ECT, sudden onset of symptoms, fluctuating course, labile mood, delusions, psychomotor retardation, prominent guilt, and early morning wakening.

H. Administration of antidepressants following successful use of ECT helps to prevent relapse. An attempt should be made to discontinue the medication 6 to 12 months after it is started. A few patients require antidepressants indefinitely.

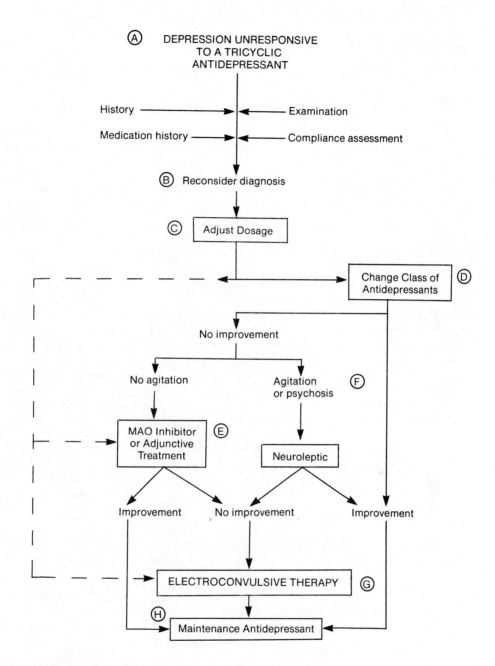

(A) DEPRESSION UNRESPONSIVE
TO A TRICYCLIC
ANTIDEPRESSANT

History ⟶ ⟵ Examination

Medication history ⟶ ⟵ Compliance assessment

(B) Reconsider diagnosis

(C) Adjust Dosage

Change Class of
Antidepressants (D)

No improvement

No agitation   Agitation
or psychosis   (F)

MAO Inhibitor (E)
or Adjunctive
Treatment

Neuroleptic

Improvement   No improvement   Improvement

ELECTROCONVULSIVE THERAPY (G)

(H) Maintenance Antidepressant

REFERENCES

Fink M. Convulsive Therapy, Theory and Practice. New York: Raven Press, 1983.
Klein EF, Gittelman R, Quitkin F, Rifkin A. Diagnosis in Drug Treatment of Psychiatric Disorders: Adults
and Children. 2nd ed. Baltimore: Williams and Wilkins, 1980.
Ayd FJ. Neuroleptics as antidepressants. Internat Drug Ther News 1983; 20: 19–20.

FIRST-LINE DRUGS USED TO TREAT DEPRESSION

Steven L. Dubovsky, M.D.

COMMENTS

A. This chapter lists first-line antidepressants now available in the United States. Administration of antidepressants should be considered in the presence of: (1) past history or family history of benefit from somatic therapy for depression, (2) vegetative signs (early morning awakening, diurnal variation of mood, anorexia, weight loss), (3) severe symptoms, (4) strongly positive family history of affective disorder, (5) positive dexamethasone suppression test (failure to suppress 4 PM or 11 PM serum cortisol below 5 μg/dl on the day after administration of 1 mg of dexamethasone at 4 PM), and (6) failure to respond to psychotherapy.

B. Antidepressants of different classes are clustered together. The first 3 classes are tricyclics; the remaining drugs have different, nontricyclic structures. Most of these first-line drugs are thought to increase brain levels of norepinephrine and serotonin to varying degrees by blocking reuptake. Amoxapine blocks reuptake of norepinephrine and dopamine, maprotiline and doxepine are primarily noradrenergic, and trazodone primarily blocks serotonin reuptake. The following may be used as basic guidelines in choosing an antidepressant: (1) The first choice is a medication to which the patient or a family member has responded in the past. (2) Trazodone and amoxapine may be safer for patients with cardiovascular disease. (3) Drugs with less prominent anticholinergic and sedating effects are safer for the elderly. (4) Amoxapine and maprotiline may aggravate epilepsy. (5) Amoxapine has a more rapid onset of action but is more likely to produce a movement disorder similar to that produced by neuroleptics. (6) Anxious, depressed patients usually receive a sedating antidepressant; patients with psychomotor slowing receive a nonsedating drug. (7) Patients who do not respond to a drug of one class are switched to a medication in another class with a presumably different primary action or neurotransmitter metabolism (e.g., from trazodone to amoxapine) or to an MAO inhibitor. (8) Priapism has recently been reported with trazodone.

C. Geriatric doses, when known, are indicated in parentheses. Pediatric doses have only been studied in imipramine. The recommended dose of this drug in children is 2.5–4.5 mg/kg/day in divided doses.

D. Imipramine, amoxapine, trazodone, alprazolam, and MAO inhibitors are also effective in the treatment of endogenous anxiety and phobias.

E. The interactions and side effects summarized may occur with any antidepressant.

REFERENCES

Grinspoon L. Depressive disorders. APA Psychiatry Update 1983; 2:354.
Electroconvulsive Therapy. Task Force Report 14. APA, Washington DC, 1978.
Klein D F, Gittelman R, Quitkin F, Rifkin A. Clinical management of affective disorders. In: Diagnosis and Drug Treatment of Psychiatric Disorders: Adults and Children. Baltimore: Williams & Wilkins, 1980.

Ⓑ Antidepressants	Ⓒ Usual Daily dose, mg	Ⓓ Special Characteristics and Indications	Ⓔ Some Interactions	Side Effects
Amitriptyline (Elavil) Nortriptyline (Aventyl) Protriptyline (Vivactyl)	150-300 (30-50) 50-150 (25-50) 10-60	More sedating Therapeutic window for nortriptyline	Interfere with action of guanethidine, clonidine and bethanedine blood levels with barbiturates and alcohol	Anticholinergic (esp.glaucoma and urinary retention) Postural hypotension
Imipramine (Tofranil) Desipramine (Pertofrane) Trimipramine (Surmontil)	150-300 (30-50) 150-250 (25-50) 50-300	May be used for panic attacks Try this class first for retarded depression or ? low 24-hour urinary MHPG Therapeutic window for desipramine Fewer autonomic side effects	Hypertension when administered with amphetamines, norepinephrine, phenylephrine, MAOIs Decreased effect of L-dopa Increased phenytoin toxicity	May precipitate heart block if preexisting bundle branch block Quinidine-like effect Weight gain Can cause impotence ? Sudden death
Doxepin (Sinequan)	75-150 (25-50)	May be less cardiotoxic		May be teratogenic (limb deformities) Excreted in breast milk; effects on newborn not known
Amoxapine (Ascendin)	150-300 (25-75)	May be less cardiotoxic; not sedating ? Somewhat faster onset of action Less anticholinergic Also blocks dopamine receptors May cause extrapyramidal side effects		
Maprotiline (Ludiomil)	150-300 (25-50)	Less anticholinergic May cause seizures		
Trazodone (Desyrel)	150-400 (50-150)	Not anticholinergic Very sedating Low cardiovascular toxicity Must be administered in divided dose		

SECOND-LINE DRUGS USED TO TREAT DEPRESSION

Steven L. Dubovsky, M.D.

COMMENTS

A. This chapter describes medications that may be effective when first-line drugs fail and drugs that are indicated for specific types of depression. The therapeutic strategy in treatment-resistant depression is outlined on pp 60–61.

B. MAO inhibitors ameliorate endogenous anxiety and atypical depression which is character-ized by lethargy, somatic complaints, self-pity, anxiety, difficulty falling asleep, worsening of symptoms at the end of the day, increased appetite, and weight gain. MAO inhibitors are probably underutilized as first-line drugs because of concomitant necessary restrictions of diet and other medications. Although MAO inhibitors are safe and effective, physician and patient should be informed about interactions with tyramine-containing foods, sympatho-mimetics, antihistamines, and other drugs.

C. Neuroleptics, with or without antidepressants, ameliorate severe anxiety, agitation, and psychotic features that accompany depression. Doses are lower than those used to treat schizophrenia and mania. As these symptoms abate, the neuroleptic should gradually be withdrawn. Because of the danger of severe anticholinergic reactions, highly anticholinergic neuroleptics such as thioridazine should not be combined with anticholinergic antidepres-sants such as amitriptyline.

D. Because amoxapine, an antidepressant, is a derivative of loxapine, the latter drug may be well suited to depression accompanied by psychosis.

E. Methylphenidate administered for about one month has been reported to improve depres-sion in some elderly and physically ill patients. Tolerance and withdrawal have not been a problem under these conditions.

F. T_3 added to tricyclics or MAOIs may enhance responsiveness to antidepressants, even if thyroid function is normal.

REFERENCES

Ayd MD, Frank J. Treatment-Resistant Depression: Therapeutic Strategies Affective Disorders Reassessed: 1983, 115-125. AYD Medical Communications, Baltimore, Maryland 1983.

Bernstein JG. Electroconvulsive therapy. In: Handbook of Drug Therapy in Psychiatry. Littleton, MA: John Wright, 1983: 115.

Bernstein JG. Monoamine oxidase inhibitors. In: Handbook of Drug Therapy in Psychiatry. Littleton, MA: John Wright, 1983: 97.

SECOND-LINE DRUGS USED TO TREAT DEPRESSION

Drug Ⓐ	Usual Daily dose	Special Characteristics and Indications	Interactions	Side Effects
MAO Inhibitors Ⓑ		Resistance to TCAs	Severe hypertension with sympathomimetics, methyldopa, tyramine-containing foods, meperidine, L-dopa; antihistamines, TCAs, many others	Anticholinergic
Phenelzine (Nardil)	60 mg	Phobic-anxiety states		Anorexia
				Weight gain
Tranylcypromine (Parnate)	20 mg	Panic attacks		Irritability, mania
		Atypical depression	Potentiation by thiazide diuretics	Impotence and anorgasmia
		Tranylcypromine only for inpatients		Postural hypotension
		Phenelzine may also be an antihypertensive		Insomnia
				Liver damage
				Infertility and fetal resorption in animals
Antipsychotics Ⓒ				
Chlorpromazine	50-300 mg	Useful in agitated depression, depression with marked anxiety or psychotic depression	May interfere with some antihypertensives	Anticholinergic
Thioridazine never give >	50-300 mg 800 mg/day		Anticholinergic side effects additive with those of antidepressants	Postural hypotension (less with haloperidol)
Haloperidol	1-10 mg			Quinidine-like effect (esp. thioridazine)
Loxapine Ⓓ	10-50 mg		Potentiation of CNS depressants by sedating antipsychotics	Parkinsonian side effects
			Phenobarbital decreases blood levels of neuroleptics	Sudden death (thioridazine)
				Tardive dyskinesia
				Impotence (thioridazine)
Stimulants Ⓔ				
Methylphenidate	10-25 mg	Useful in elderly and medically ill patients	Dangerous hypertension when administered concurrently with MAOIs or tricyclics	Drug dependence rare in depressed medical patients
Other adjuncts				
Ⓕ T₃ (Cytomel)	25-50 µg	May enhance responsiveness to TCAs, especially in women	May be safely combined with MAOIs	
L-Tryptophan Pyrodoxine (Vit. B₆)	4-15 g/ 200/mg	Serotonergic (B₆ is a necessary cofactor)		

NEW ANTIDEPRESSANTS

Steven L. Dubovsky, M.D.

COMMENTS

A. Newer antidepressants produce fewer anticholinergic and cardiotoxic side effects. Some do not fit the catecholamine hypothesis of depression in that they do not affect reuptake of norepinephrine (NE) or serotonin (5–HT).

B. Mianserin blocks alpha-2 and histamine H_2 receptors but does not affect reuptake of NE or 5–HT. It is relatively safe when taken in overdose and has low cardiovascular toxicity; however, it may prove to be associated with agranulocytosis.

C. Fluoxetine potentiates 5-HT without affecting NE or dopamine (DA) metabolism. It has low anticholinergic toxicity and may be especially useful for retarded depression.

D. Zimelidine is a 5-HT reuptake inhibitor. It has low cardiovascular toxicity, has no anticholinergic effects, and does not produce weight gain.

E. Fluvoxamine inhibits 5–HT reuptake without affecting DA, NE, or monoamine oxidase (MAO) activity. It has minimal cardiovascular and anticholinergic effects.

F. Bupropion is associated with weight loss rather than gain. It has been used most effectively in the treatment of retarded depression in adolescents. Its primary effect is on DA reuptake; it is not anticholinergic.

G. Nomifensine inhibits reuptake of NE and DA. It is not sedating or cardiotoxic, is safe when taken in overdose, and does not lower the seizure threshold. However, it has demonstrated amphetamine-like properties that are not related to release of catecholamines.

REFERENCES

Hollister LE. Clinical Use of Psychotherapeutic Drugs. 2nd ed. Springfield, Illinois: CC Thomas, 1981.
Klein DF, Gittelman R, Quitkin F, Rifkin A. Diagnosis and Drug Treatment of Psychiatric Disorders: Adults and Children. 2nd ed. Baltimore: Williams & Wilkins, 1980.

Ⓐ NEW ANTIDEPRESSANTS NOT YET RELEASED IN THE U.S.

Drug	Type	Probable Daily Dose
Ⓑ Mianserin	tetracyclic	30 – 150 mg
Ⓒ Fluoxetine	bicyclic	40 – 80 mg
Ⓓ Zimelidine	bicyclic	100 – 300 mg
Ⓔ Fluvoxamine	unicyclic	50 – 300 mg
Ⓕ Bupropion	unicyclic	200 – 600 mg
Ⓖ Nomifensine	heterocyclic	100 – 200 mg

ANTIANXIETY DRUGS

Steven L. Dubovsky, M.D.

COMMENTS

A. Because they produce drug dependence, addiction, and dangerous abstinence syndromes and are lethal when taken in overdose, barbiturates, glycerol derivatives, and related drugs are no longer used as tranquilizers and sedatives. Methaqualone (Quaalude) was recently withdrawn from the market.

B. Benzodiazepines are generally effective and safe. Fatalities after overdosage are rare in patients taking 700 mg/day who do not also ingest another substance such as alcohol. Addiction is rare when these drugs are used under medical supervision. Abstinence syndromes may occur up to 2 weeks after discontinuing the drug in patients taking >40-60 mg/day of diazepam or its equivalent. Withdrawal syndrome has been reported with lower doses. Blood levels of diazepam and chlordiazepoxide, but not lorazepam, are increased by cimetidine. Concerns about teratogenicity of diazepam (cleft palate, limb deformities) have been overstated. In addition to its antianxiety properties, alprazolam may ameliorate panic attacks and some depressions.

C. Because they do not produce drug dependence, the sedating effects of antihistamines may be used to reduce anxiety in addiction-prone patients. However, anxiety reduction is less predictable than with benzodiazepines. Antihistamines are also used as hypnotics in the elderly.

D. Propranolol can be administered to anxious patients with marked tremor and tachycardia. It is also useful for stage fright. High doses may decrease unpredictable violent outbursts in some demented patients.

REFERENCES

Antianxiety drugs, sleeping pills, insomnia, and medical practice. Institute of Medicine, Division of Mental Health and Behavioral Medicine, National Academy of Sciences, 1979.
Gilman AG, Goodman LS, Gilman A. The Pharmacological Basis of Therapeutics. New York: Macmillan, 1980.

(A) **ANTIANXIETY DRUGS**

	Examples	Usual daily dose, mg
(B) Benzodiazepines	diazepam (Valium)	4–20 mg
	chlordiazepoxide (Librium)	20–100 mg
	chlorazepate (Tranxene)	15–22.5 mg
	oxazepam (Serax)	30–45 mg
	lorazepam (Ativan)	1–10 mg
	alprazolam (Xanax)	1.5–6 mg
	flurazepam (Dalmane)	15–30 mg
	temazepam (Restoril)	15–30 mg
	triazolam (Halcion)	0.25–0.75 mg
(C) Sedative autonomic antihistamines	hydroxyzine (Atarax)	100–200 mg
	diphenyhydramine (Benadryl)	100–200 mg
(D) Beta-blocking agents	propranolol (Inderal)	40–120 mg

ATYPICAL PHYSICAL SYMPTOMS

Carl J. Getto, M.D.

COMMENTS

A. A complete psychiatric differential diagnosis of the unexplained somatic complaint, and factors suggesting functional overlay are outlined on pp 84–85. This chapter describes a general approach to unclear psychosomatic syndromes. When psychiatric consultation is requested, the patient should be reassured that the primary physician will not abandon him. A return appointment with the primary physician should be scheduled before the patient sees the psychiatrist.

B. Often, some but not all of the patient's symptoms can be explained by an identifiable pathophysiologic process. In pursuing the medical evaluation, appropriate restraint is necessary in order to avoid uncovering minor abnormalities that could become a focus for further complaints.

C. Psychiatric diagnoses should not be suggested solely because a medical disorder cannot be specified. If no positive signs of a psychiatric condition likely to be associated with somatic complaints are present, the patient's problem should be assumed to be physical until proven otherwise.

D. "Masked depression" presents with vague, generalized, or atypical physical complaints rather than emotional symptoms. A past history of depression or treatment for depression, a family history of affective disorder or alcoholism, and a positive dexamethasone suppression test, are useful clues that physical complaints are caused by depression. Careful questioning may reveal altered mood, feelings of worthlessness, hopelessness, decreased self-esteem, and vegetative signs. Antidepressants may be indicated even if depression cannot be confirmed. Improvement may be measured by better functioning, improved mood, and decreased vegetative signs rather than by abatement of original physical complaint.

E. A careful history may reveal a past psychosis. Detailed questioning about current symptoms may reveal bizarre, idiosyncratic, or paranoid ideas indicating that the patient is attempting to control psychotic thoughts by focusing on minor physiologic dysfunctions.

F. Delirious and demented patients may use physical complaints to distract themselves from cognitive or memory defects. Many somatizing patients take multiple drugs, particularly tranquilizers, hypnotics, and analgesics; the most likely cause of organic brain syndrome in a patient with longstanding physical complaints is intoxication with, or withdrawal from centrally acting compounds. If irreversible dementia (pp 98–99) is found after all drugs are withdrawn, CNS depressants should be avoided. Usually the patient must be assured of an ongoing relationship with the physician before he will agree to discontinue medications to which he is emotionally attached.

G. Physical complaints may be used to avoid responsibilities or conflicts, to gain attention, or to cement a failing relationship. Family or marital therapy is necessary to address the reasons why interpersonal problems cannot be addressed more directly.

H. Somatoform disorders are characterized by physical complaints influenced by psychological factors, and not due to any identifiable pathophysiologic process or to another major psychiatric disorder. Diagnostic categories include somatization disorder (hysteria or Briquet's syndrome), psychogenic pain disorder, and hypochondriasis, which are treated similarly and conversion disorder (conversion hysteria).

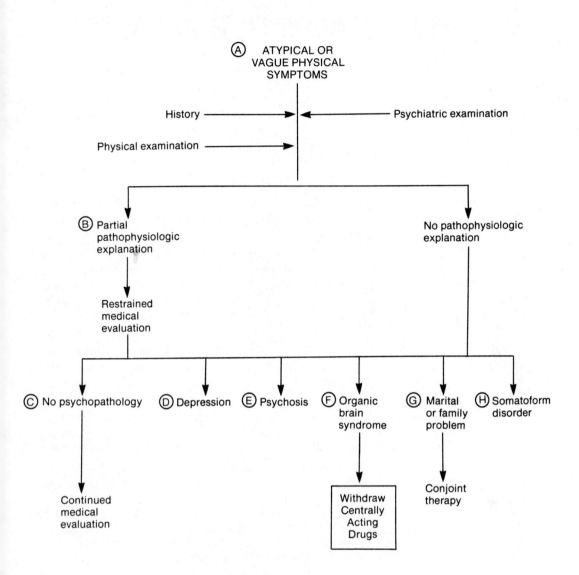

A ATYPICAL OR
VAGUE PHYSICAL
SYMPTOMS

History ⟶ ⟵ Psychiatric examination

Physical examination ⟶

B Partial
pathophysiologic
explanation

No pathophysiologic
explanation

Restrained
medical
evaluation

C No psychopathology D Depression E Psychosis F Organic
brain
syndrome

G Marital
or family
problem

H Somatoform
disorder

Continued
medical
evaluation

Withdraw
Centrally
Acting
Drugs

Conjoint
therapy

REFERENCES

Greist JH, Jefferson JW, Spitzer RL, eds. Treatment of Mental Disorders. New York: Oxford University
Press, 1982: 387–397.
Engel GL. "Psychogenic" pain and the pain-prone patient. Amer J Med 1959; 26:899–918.

BENIGN INTRACTABLE PAIN
Carl J. Getto, M.D.

COMMENTS

A. Chronic pain not due to neoplastic disease or other severe physical disease may be a stable complaint, it may change over time, or it may be relapsing, with exacerbations at time of stress. Symptoms usually begin after an injury or illness from which the patient does not recover as expected. Standard medical and surgical treatments may produce some initial relief, but improvement is only transient. The typical patient with benign intractable pain demonstrates constricted emotional functioning, inability to verbalize emotions, and impoverished interpersonal relations. Pain, which increases at times of stress, becomes the central focus of the patient's thoughts, behavior and relationships. Any suggestion that psychological forces play a role arouses anxiety and anger.

B. Intensive therapy is indicated for patients who are motivated to relinquish this means of dealing with stress. Sufficient psychological flexibility is indicated by (1) symptom duration <2 years without previous prolonged episodes of physical incapacitation; (2) willingness of patient and family to engage in intensive treatment; (3) absence of major psychiatric disorder other than depression; (4) history of success in work and interpersonal relationships.

C. Dependence on multiple drugs, especially opioids, tranquilizers, and sleeping pills may confuse the picture and lead to continued complaints in order to maintain medication levels that will prevent abstinence symptoms. Remission or decreased complaints may result from withdrawal of all centrally acting drugs.

D. If an injury is work- or accident-related, compensation may be contingent on continuing complaints. It is unrealistic to expect the patient to relinquish behavior that results in financial reward. If unsettled litigation cannot be resolved before treatment proceeds, the physician who evaluates disability should not be the physician who initiates psychotherapy.

E. Aggressive treatment of chronic pain has 4 components: (1) An individualized physical therapy program begins with activities the patient can accomplish and proceeds in graduated steps. The patient is allowed to rest only when he has completed an activity, not when he complains or protests incapacity. (2) Healthy, nonpain behavior such as going to work, staying out of bed, and not taking medication, is rewarded with attention, praise, rest, or other gains the patient has identified as positive; pain behavior such as discussing symptoms, refusing to work, or avoiding social responsibilities is ignored. (3) Psychotherapy and antidepressants are prescribed for suspected depression. (4) The family is taught to identify and administer rewards for nonpain behavior and to stop providing covert encouragement for pain behavior. Unresolved family conflicts that maintain patient impairment must be addressed by the entire family.

F. Even if symptoms remit completely, ongoing follow-up is necessary to monitor stresses to which the patient may respond with increased complaints and to reassure the patient that he does not have to be in pain to have continuing relationships.

G. Inability to adopt a less impaired role is suggested by: long-standing symptoms, a need to use pain as an excuse for shortcomings, the expectation that caretaking is owed the patient because he is sick, prominent anger, hostility and aggression, and a family that wants the patient to remain ill.

H. Supportive psychotherapy provides *care* rather than *cure*. Its goal is to maintain functioning in spite of symptoms rather than to remove symptoms. Principles of treatment include: (1)avoidance of challenges to the patient's claim to be ill; (2) regularly scheduled, time-limited appointments that continue indefinitely even if the patient improves; (3) discussion of the patient's reactions to his symptoms rather than the causes of his symptoms; and (4)judicious use of nonaddicting medications.

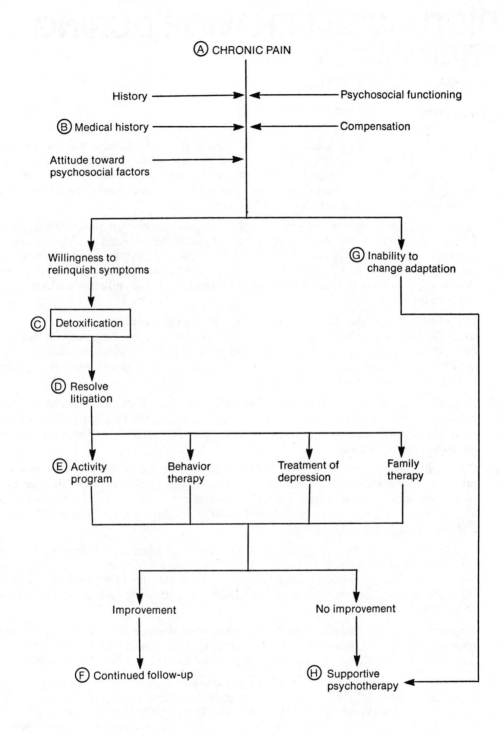

REFERENCES

Fordyce W. Behavioral Methods for Chronic Pain and Illness. St. Louis: CV Mosby, 1976.
Greist JH, Jefferson JW, Spitzer RL, eds. Treatment of Mental Disorders. New York: Oxford University
    Press, 1982: 277–286.

DISTURBED BEHAVIOR DURING PREGNANCY

Janice Petersen, M.D.

COMMENTS

A. Baseline data include patient and family psychiatric history, difficulties in previous pregnancies and interventions that were helpful, available supports, relationship with the father of the child, conflicts about the pregnancy, financial status and life situation. Pregnancy is associated with increased feelings of dependency; the doctor's attitude and the patient's feelings about him can have great impact on her behavior.

B. Latent psychoses are precipitated in 0.1 to 0.2% of pregnant women; these are likely to be affective disorders, schizoaffective disorders, or rarely, schizophrenia. Neuroleptics are generally safe during pregnancy; lithium is definitely and tricyclic antidepressants and antianxiety drugs are probably teratogenic; monoamine oxidase inhibitors cause fetal resorption in animals. Most psychotropic drugs are excreted in breast milk; their effects on the newborn are unknown.

C. Disturbed behavior during pregnancy often occurs in the context of disruption in the patient's relationships with the father of the child, her parents or other supportive figures, or a disrupted social situation. Interventions to correct social problems include meetings with the family to discuss conflicts, assistance with shelter, food, and finances, and visiting nurse service to provide education and structure.

D. Pregnancy does not convey any special protection against self-destructive behavior; such behavior should be evaluated as in any potentially suicidal patient. Pregnant patients who are harmful to themselves are also at higher risk for child abuse; suicidal acts may represent an attempt to injure the child.

E. Chronically disorganized patients who find it difficult to follow through with necessary prenatal treatment benefit from a concrete plan that is firmly insisted upon by the physician, frequent reminders about appointments, and aggressive outreach by the physician and visiting nurses. Any existing supports (family, friends, teachers, neighbors) should be identified and strengthened.

F. Patients who become excessively angry during pregnancy often are attempting to control fears of being too dependent on the physician by gaining greater emotional distance from him. Allowing the patient as much control as possible over treatment, respecting her wish for independence, and deferring to her when possible may increase feelings of security and decrease anger.

G. Pregnant patients who become excessively dependent need to be encouraged to assume more responsibility for themselves. Regular, frequent appointments should be scheduled, while unscheduled calls and unannounced visits to the physician or clinic should be limited.

H. Pregnant patients should be advised not to consume any alcohol at all or definitely less than 3 oz in a day. The use of all psychoactive drugs during pregnancy should be strictly limited and treatment prescribed early for drug abusers. Narcotic withdrawal late in pregnancy is probably more dangerous to the fetus than maintenance with methadone; babies born to narcotic-dependent mothers will experience a postnatal abstinence syndrome.

REFERENCES

Dubovsky SL. Psychiatric approach to high-risk obstetrics. In: Abrams R, Wexler P, eds. Medical Complications in Obstetrics. Boston: Little, Brown, 1983.

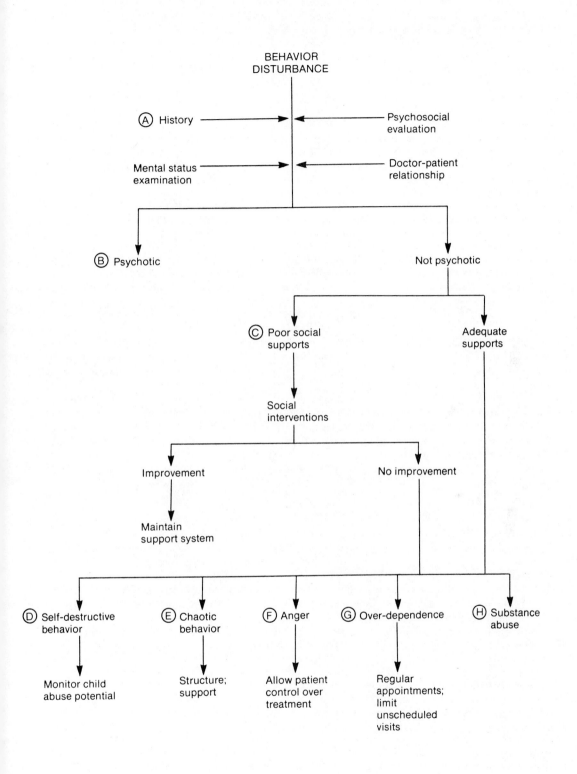

BEHAVIOR
DISTURBANCE

Ⓐ History

Psychosocial
evaluation

Mental status
examination

Doctor-patient
relationship

Ⓑ Psychotic

Not psychotic

Ⓒ Poor social
supports

Adequate
supports

Social
interventions

Improvement

No improvement

Maintain
support system

Ⓓ Self-destructive
behavior

Ⓔ Chaotic
behavior

Ⓕ Anger

Ⓖ Over-dependence

Ⓗ Substance
abuse

Monitor child
abuse potential

Structure;
support

Allow patient
control over
treatment

Regular
appointments;
limit
unscheduled
visits

Hatherly L. Psychiatric disorders in obstetrics. Obstet Gynecol Survey 1980; 35:439–441.
Daly MJ. The emotional problems of patients encountered in the practice of obstetrics and gynecology.
    Obstet Gynecol Annual 1980; 9:339–356.

THE DYING PATIENT

Janice Petersen, M.D.

COMMENTS

A. The patient's understanding of the illness and its treatment, previous level of functioning, past psychiatric history, coping style, the symbolic meaning of the illness, the family's reaction, and the presence of depression or organic brain disease all influence adjustment to a terminal illness.

B. Feelings of failure, detachment, or overinvolvement may interfere with the physician's ability to be consistently available emotionally and to allow the patient as much control as possible over the treatment.

C. Patients experiencing severe pain may need very high doses of narcotic analgesics; they may benefit from medications that augment analgesia such as phenothiazines and antidepressants. Hypnosis may be a useful adjunct, but adequate pain relief remains the primary goal.

D. Psychological "stages" of dying (denial, anger, bargaining, depression and acceptance) are in part manifestations of grief (pp 54–55) over loss of health, functioning, and the impending loss of all loved ones. The family often needs help with their mourning, as well.

E. Unless the patient prefers to confront his illness alone, the family should be involved in the patient's treatment and encouraged to be available to the patient. The family may need help with their grief over the forthcoming loss of the patient.

F. The involvement of family members in longstanding conflict with the patient may need to be limited and other supportive family members and friends mobilized. Avoidance of the patient or denial of the seriousness of his illness may be due to fear of experiencing grief, in which case empathic support may help them begin mourning. If the family has already mourned but the patient has not yet died, they may have given up their emotional investment in the patient and become incapable of reestablishing attachment to him. Support and education about the grieving process may help to relieve their guilt over not being available to the patient; the physician and others may need to be more available, to compensate for the family's unavailability.

G. If the patient is compliant and making appropriate plans, denial (pp 4–5) should not be challenged if it helps decrease anxiety.

H. Apparent emotional withdrawal may be caused by inanition or excessive dosage of medications. When the patient is resigned to death and gradually withdrawing, the family and medical staff may need education about this adaptive behavior and encouragement to continue their involvement, even though the patient is not as responsive as he once was. Depression is distinguished from other forms of withdrawal by the presence of anger, guilt, worthlessness, tearfulness, and a sense of unfulfilled tasks.

I. Dying patients may be angry with physicians for not curing them and with family and friends for being healthy, or they may use anger to avoid sadness about dying and anxiety about loss of control. Ventilating feelings of disappointment, addressing realistic complaints, allowing the patient as much control as possible over his care, and limiting disruptive behavior may help him control negative reactions.

J. Panic about dying may reflect fears of being helpless, in pain, or alone. Visitors, complete information about the proposed treatment, pain relief, and antianxiety medication usually decrease intense anxiety.

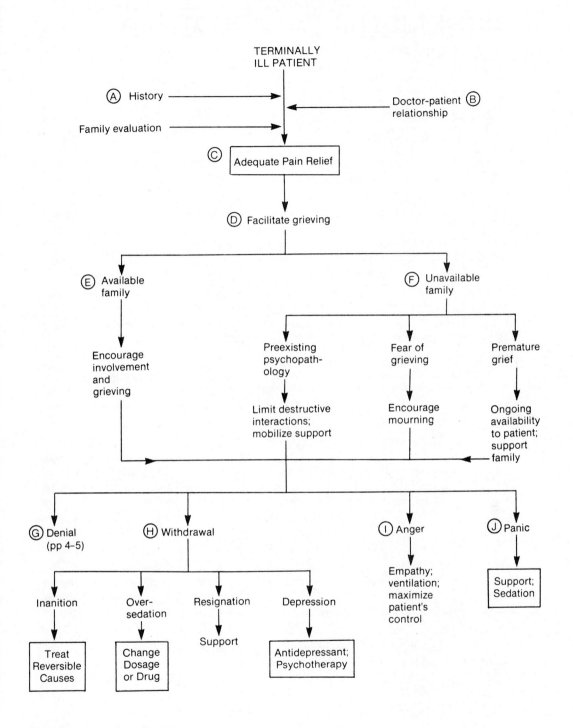

TERMINALLY
ILL PATIENT

(A) History ⟶ ⟵ Doctor-patient (B)
relationship

Family evaluation ⟶

(C) Adequate Pain Relief

(D) Facilitate grieving

(E) Available family

(F) Unavailable family

Encourage
involvement
and
grieving

Preexisting
psychopath-
ology

Fear of
grieving

Premature
grief

Limit destructive
interactions;
mobilize support

Encourage
mourning

Ongoing
availability
to patient;
support
family

(G) Denial
(pp 4–5)

(H) Withdrawal

(I) Anger

(J) Panic

Inanition

Over-
sedation

Resignation

Depression

Empathy;
ventilation;
maximize
patient's
control

Support;
Sedation

Treat
Reversible
Causes

Change
Dosage
or Drug

Support

Antidepressant;
Psychotherapy

REFERENCES

Kubler-Ross E. On Death and Dying. New York: Macmillan, 1969.
Pasnau RO, ed. Consultation-Liaison Psychiatry. New York: Grune & Stratton, 1975.
Hackett TP, Cassem NH. Handbook of General Hospital Psychiatry. St. Louis: CV Mosby, 1978.

HYPEREMESIS GRAVIDARUM

Janice Petersen, M.D.

COMMENTS

A. At least some nausea and vomiting occurs in the first trimester in 50 to 80% of otherwise normal pregnancies. "Morning sickness" probably has a *physiological* etiology; it is hyperemesis gravidarum when vomiting is severe enough to warrant hospitalization. Hyperemesis is often associated with conflicts about the pregnancy and family problems in addition to physiologic factors. It is difficult to determine the degree to which ambivalence about the pregnancy causes or results from pathological vomiting.

B. History should focus on the circumstances of the pregnancy, the patient's relationships with the father of the child and with her parents, feelings about the pregnancy, experiences with previous pregnancies, and available supports. Examine for dehydration, weight loss, and other possible consequences of vomiting. Baseline laboratory studies include BUN, serum electrolytes and urinary ketones.

C. Intractable vomiting can lead to retarded fetal growth, and severe maternal morbidity and mortality. Intravenous hydration is essential. The patient should be admitted to a single room; psychosocial stimulation should be limited. Antiemetics may be prescribed although vomiting usually stops spontaneously after a few days.

D. When the social situation is chaotic or disrupted, family therapy to resolve conflicts, especially with the father of the child and the patient's mother, may help to reduce emotional distress that contributes to vomiting. If the immediate family and husband are not available or are unsupportive, other supports such as grandparents, friends, social service or visiting nurses should be identified.

E. Conflicts with important people, mixed feelings about the pregnancy and a wish to avoid responsibility are psychological factors in hyperemesis. The patient has little if any insight into these issues and is not equipped emotionally to resolve them. Psychodynamic psycho-therapy is therefore avoided. All stresses are withdrawn, visiting is restricted, and the patient is temporarily made dependent to allow her to mobilize her defenses. Responsibility and relationships are then reintroduced at a pace the patient can tolerate. Hypnosis, with suggestions of relaxation, calm and well-being, is a useful adjunct if manipulation of social relationships alone is unsuccessful. It reduces symptoms in more than 60% of patients.

F. If the patient's dependency needs are transferred to the physician through frequent prenatal visits, there may be less pressure to seek caretaking through vomiting and other physical symptoms. Neither the patient nor the physician should be surprised or dismayed if vomiting returns; it is likely to remit quickly following rehospitalization and repeat of the maneuvers outlined above.

G. Extended hospitalization and behavior therapy is necessary if vomiting does not respond to supportive care and hypnosis. Visitors are restricted and vomiting ignored; the nursing staff's attention is focused on eating, self-care and weight gain. Visits and other rewards are permitted only when the patient stops vomiting.

REFERENCES

Fairweather D. Nausea and vomiting in pregnancy. Amer J Obstet Gynecol 1968; 102:135–175.

Fuchs K, Paldi E, Abramovici H, et al. Treatment of hyperemesis gravidarum by hypnosis. Internat J Clin Exp Hypn 1980; 28:313–328.

Katon WJ, Kies R. Hyperemesis gravidarum: a biopsychosocial perspective. Internat J Psychiatry Med 1980; 10:151–162.

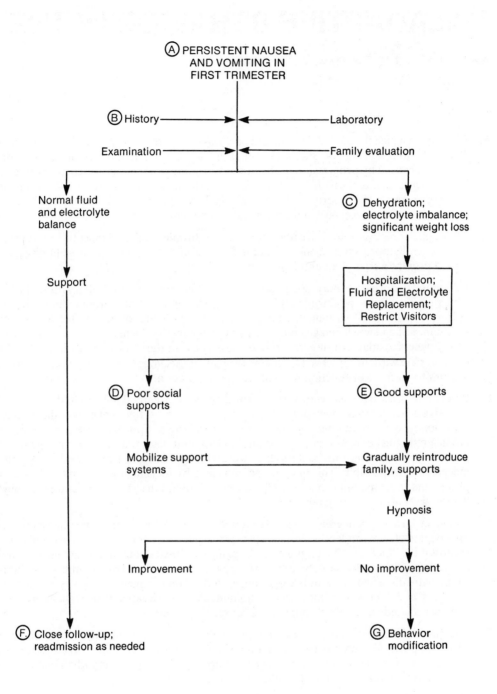

MALADAPTIVE BEHAVIOR IN THE CHRONICALLY ILL

Janice Petersen, M.D.

COMMENTS

A. The ways in which the patient has handled previous stress predict how he will adapt to current illness. A thorough mental status examination is necessary to exclude an organic brain syndrome caused by progression of the illness or by *any* drug administered in chronic care. Psychological dysfunction often reflects physical disability, interference with daily functioning, or disruption of supportive relations or social/occupational functioning. Evaluation of suicide potential is necessary in all chronically ill patients.

B. Although depressive feelings are ubiquitous in the chronically ill and must be treated as part of the overall approach, evidence of major depression or a strongly positive family history should prompt a trial of an antidepressant.

C. Behavioral disturbances may be due to reluctance to accept irreversible illness or to difficulty adjusting to life as a chronically ill patient. Acceptance of chronic illness involves acknowledgement of permanent changes in the patient's life, mourning for lost abilities, acceptance of a new self-image, and a new role in the family. Denial, inadequate mourning, unwillingness to adapt, or discomfort in the family about the changes necessitated by illness may interfere with this process. Discussing the patient's feelings about being ill and encouraging him to mourn lost functioning facilitate his adaptation.

D. Illness may lead patients who were deprived of normal caretaking in childhood to seek excessive dependency through preoccupation with symptoms, frequent calls to the physician, demanding behavior, and inappropriate reliance on others. Appropriate dependency on the physician should be encouraged by regular, brief appointments that are not contingent on the patient demonstrating incapacitation; however, the patient must be helped to remain as independent as possible. This may be accomplished by focusing discussions on his accomplishments and remaining abilities while paying less attention to the illness and expecting the highest level of functioning possible.

E. Patients who fear any degree of dependency may avoid acknowledging their illness and insist on a degree of independence of which they are incapable. They may feel a greater sense of control if the illness and its treatment are explained in great detail, if they are given as much choice as possible in decisions regarding therapy, and if the physician accommodates himself to the patient's schedule. Ventilation of anger and disappointment, emphasis on remaining strengths, and discussion of the patient's thoughts about the treatment also relieve pressure to demonstrate independence through inappropriate behavior.

F. If disturbed behavior represents an attempt to call the physician's attention to an absence of social supports, visiting nurse services, day care programs, activities by organizations concerned with the patient's illness, and group therapy with other patients with the same disease decrease isolation and help to structure the patient's life.

G. While the physician spends little time with the patient, the family must deal with him day in and day out. Family therapy can be extremely helpful in elucidating reactions to changing roles and covert encouragement of psychiatric symptoms, and in teaching the family new ways of interacting with the patient.

REFERENCES

Krupp N. Adaptation to chronic illness. Postgraduate Medicine 1976; 60:122–125.

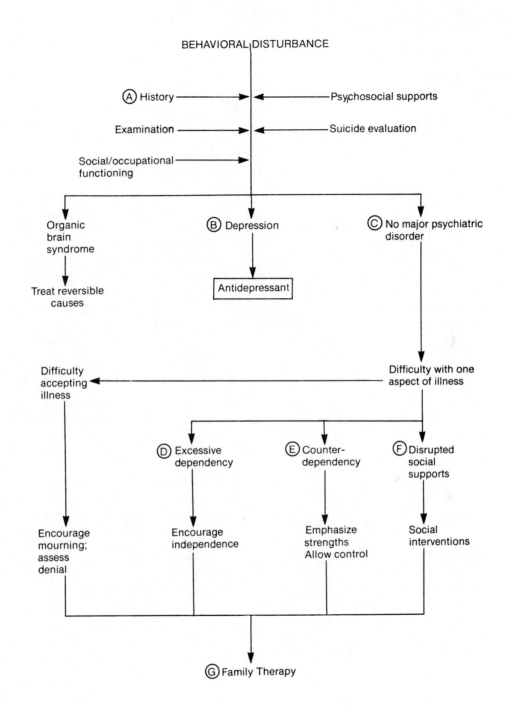

BEHAVIORAL DISTURBANCE

(A) History ⟶ ⟵ Psychosocial supports

Examination ⟶ ⟵ Suicide evaluation

Social/occupational ⟶
functioning

Organic
brain
syndrome

(B) Depression

(C) No major psychiatric
disorder

Treat reversible
causes

Antidepressant

Difficulty
accepting
illness

Difficulty with one
aspect of illness

(D) Excessive
dependency

(E) Counter-
dependency

(F) Disrupted
social
supports

Encourage
mourning;
assess
denial

Encourage
independence

Emphasize
strengths
Allow control

Social
interventions

(G) Family Therapy

Levy NL. The chronically ill patient. Psychiatric Quart 1979; 51:189–197.
Strain JJ. Psychological reactions to chronic medical illness. Psychiatric Quart 1979; 51:173–183.
Lipowski ZJ. Physical illness, the individual and the coping process. Psychiatry Med 1970; 1:91–102.

SECONDARY GAIN

Carl J. Getto, M.D.

COMMENTS

A. Secondary gains are concrete, tangible benefits derived from being sick, such as exemption from responsibility, attention, gratification of dependency needs, and financial compensation. In contrast, primary gain is the unconscious benefit of solving or relieving an intrapsychic problem through developing a physical symptom. Many psychiatric disorders characterized by prominent physical complaints are maintained by both primary and secondary gain. Many bona fide medical problems produce secondary gain; this gain should not be assumed to cause the patient's symptoms. Suspicion that secondary gain is an important factor in maintaining physical symptoms is raised by: excessive complaints after an accident or industrial injury; multiple insurance, disability and compensation forms presented to the physician by the patient; calls from the patient's attorney; manifest concern about symptoms that is not as great as the extent of disability might suggest; reluctance to participate in appropriate treatment; inconsistent symptoms that do not fit known physiologic patterns; history of similar symptoms for obvious gain.

B. Conversion symptoms reflect an unconscious psychological conflict and are not under voluntary control. Common manifestations include neurological symptoms, autonomic or endocrine disturbances, vomiting, and glomus hystericus (lump in the throat that prevents swallowing), and pseudocyesis. Conversion symptoms usually appear suddenly in response to an acute emotional stress and resolve rapidly without treatment. Most patients resist psychological insight.

C. Situations in which disability is produced or maintained by compensation are characterized by a mixture of conscious and unconscious motivations. Primary gain in the form of meeting dependency needs of which the patient is unaware usually accompany secondary gain in the form of money. Litigation and disability status must be resolved before any treatment plan can be successful (pp 72–73).

D. Malingering is the voluntary simulation of physical illness to obtain obviously secondary gain such as money, drugs, or avoidance of legal sanctions. In contrast, factitious disorder (Munchausen's syndrome) is conscious simulation of disease for no gain other than to be a patient. Malingering is a sign of dishonesty rather than a specific disorder, and is generally overdiagnosed. Signs of malingering include: grossly exaggerated symptoms, lack of cooperation with diagnostic procedures, loss of symptoms when the patient is enjoying himself or is not being observed, history of similar symptoms being "cured" when secondary gain obtained, threatening behavior, and antisocial personality disorder (pp 138–139).

E. The patient should be told that his workup is negative and that his illness will probably resolve with time and conservative management. He may be helped to maintain self-esteem if he is not immediately confronted strongly. Patients with some psychoses and severe personality disorders simulate symptoms of physical disease in order to feel they are in control of some aspect of their functioning. Patients who produce symptoms only for conscious gain should be referred to an agency that is more likely to meet their needs; the physician should refuse to prescribe tranquilizers, sedatives or hypnotics.

REFERENCES

Ford CV. The Somatizing Disorders: Illness as a Way of Life. New York: Elsevier, 1983.
Lipsett DR. Psychodynamic considerations of hypochondriasis. Psychother Psychosom 1974; 23:132–136.

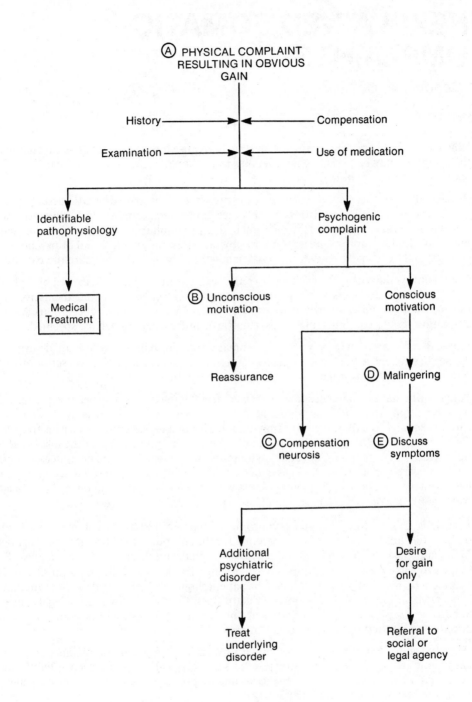

UNEXPLAINED SOMATIC COMPLAINTS

Deborah A. Coyle, M.D.

COMMENTS

A. When a careful history and examination reveal no cause for a persistent physical compliant, the symptom may be psychogenic. The physician should convey concern regardless of the etiology of the complaint.

B. Physical distress may be psychogenic in the presence of: bizarre, dramatic descriptions of symptoms; exaggeration of distress; appearance of new symptoms as old complaints resolving; symptoms of equal intensity in different body sites simultaneously; clear secondary gains; highly symbolic symptoms in response to obvious stress; adamant denial of psychological conflict; and the conviction that the physician is the only one who can cure the patient.

C. Complaints with functional overlay may reflect exaggeration of distress caused by a physiologic disturbance. Patients with organic brain syndromes frequently distract themselves from the underlying cognitive deficit by focusing attention on minor bodily aberrations. Medical evaluation should continue unless a psychiatric disorder can definitely be specified.

D. Physical complaints may be caused by somatic (haptic) halluncinations or delusions of disease in schizophrenic or psychotically depressed patients. The patient's description of the cause of his symptoms usually reveals psychotic thoughts.

E. Patients who have experienced an unexpected, frightening illness may become preoccupied with symptoms that they fear signal recurrence. They are usually reassured when, after careful examination, they are told firmly that this is not a repeat episode. Grief is frequently accompanied by diffuse aches, pains and symptoms that mimic those of the lost loved one (identification symptoms). Conversion symptoms, (the conversion of an unconscious conflict into physical complaints) are highly symbolic of underlying conflict, result in secondary gain, occur in a patient known to respond to stress with somatic symptoms, and may be associated with relative unconcern about the complaint (pp 82–83).

F. Factitious disorder (Munchausen's syndrome) is characterized by the voluntary production of dramatic, unlikely, symptoms, apparently for the sole purpose of becoming an inpatient. Munchausen patients often have had repeated hospitalizations under different names. They frequently leave the hospital abruptly when presented with negative findings (pp 82–83). The treatment of this condition is unknown; the patient should be encouraged to discuss his illness further. Malingerers, who consciously simulate illness for obvious financial or legal gain tend to become angry when their symptoms are not verified. They should be confronted more directly and referred to the appropriate agency.

G. Anxiety (pp 52–53) may be associated with generalized physical complaints and signs of autonomic arousal. Hyperventilation produces neurological symptoms such as lightheadedness, headache, blurred vision, paresthesias and carpopedal spasm. Acute episodes may be terminated by breathing into a paper bag.

H. Depressed and hypochondriacal patients both may have chronic physical complaints with similar presentations. If the patient avoids physicians, or describes vegetative or other possible signs of depression (pp 46–47), he should be treated as if depressed. Because the hypochondriac seeks to prove how sick he is in order to obtain caretaking in the form of an ongoing relationship with a physician, his complaints increase when he is threatened by not being considered ill (illness-seeking behavior) and decrease when he is reassured that he is really sick (pg. 46-47). An appropriate trial of an antidepressant tends to improve physical complaints caused by depression; hypochondriacal symptoms diminish somewhat initially but eventually return along with complaints that the medication is no longer effective.

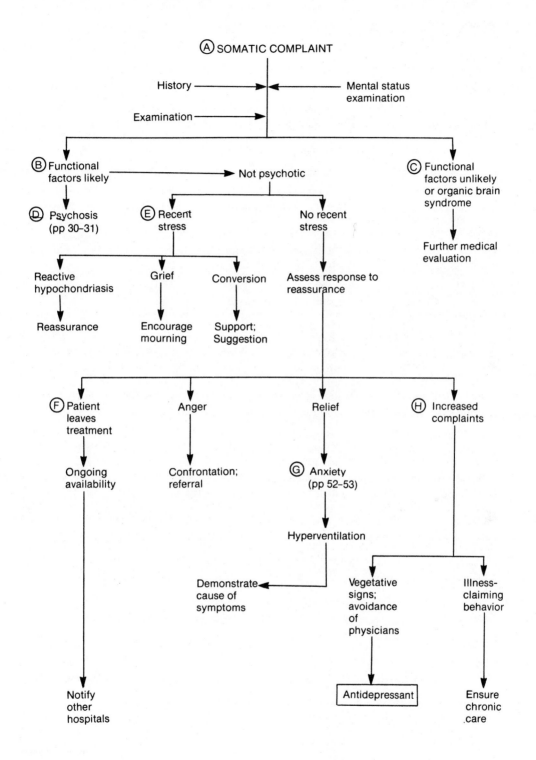

(A) SOMATIC COMPLAINT

History ──────→ ←────── Mental status examination

Examination ──────→

(B) Functional factors likely ──────→ Not psychotic

(C) Functional factors unlikely or organic brain syndrome

↓ Further medical evaluation

(D) Psychosis (pp 30–31)

(E) Recent stress

No recent stress

Reactive hypochondriasis

↓ Reassurance

Grief

↓ Encourage mourning

Conversion

↓ Support; Suggestion

Assess response to reassurance

(F) Patient leaves treatment

↓ Ongoing availability

Anger

↓ Confrontation; referral

Relief

↓ (G) Anxiety (pp 52–53)

↓ Hyperventilation

(H) Increased complaints

Demonstrate cause of symptoms ←──

Vegetative signs; avoidance of physicians

Illness-claiming behavior

↓ Notify other hospitals

↓ Antidepressant

↓ Ensure chronic care

REFERENCES

Dubovsky SL, Weissberg MP. Clinical Psychiatry in Primary Care. 2nd ed. Baltimore: Williams & Wilkins, 1982.
Dewsbury AR. Hypochondriasis and Disease-claiming Behavior in General Practice. J Royal Coll Gen Pract 1973; 23:379–383.

BAD DREAMS

Eric Haddes, Ph.D.

COMMENTS

A. Baseline history includes review of major stresses, body movements and screaming during sleep, progression of symptoms, use of medications, alcohol, and nonprescription drugs, and psychiatric symptoms during the day.

B. Sleep terrors are characterized by screams, thrashing, and elevated pulse and blood pressure. The patient does not remember the dream. Sleep terrors may accompany post-traumatic stress disorder (pp 52–53), in which anxiety, depression, preoccupation with a traumatic event, insomnia, and disturbance of psychosocial functioning persist more than 3 months after the trauma has abated. Helping the patient to relive the event in order to gain a greater sense of control over it decreases the pressure to reexperience the trauma in sleep. Diazepam, imipramine or an MAO inhibitor may decrease night terrors.

C. Sleep terrors and sleepwalking may accompany any febrile illness. Evidence of nocturnal seizures, such as tongue biting, enuresis or teeth clenching (pp 88–89), warrants a neurological investigation, since paroxysmal night terrors may result from temporal lobe epilepsy.

D. In contrast with night terrors, nightmares (dream anxiety attacks) are not accompanied by sustained vocalization, body movements, or signs of autonomic arousal. The patient is likely to remember the dream if he wakens soon afterwards, although memory the next day may be vague. Nightmares are common in children and are usually benign. In adults, they often indicate serious psychopathology. Nightmares may be caused by tricyclic antidepressants administered in one *hs* dose, alcohol withdrawal, and amphetamines.

E. If there is no precipitating stress or psychological conflict, sleep terrors and nightmares are often self-limited. However, if symptoms are progressive, insight-oriented psychotherapy may be necessary to discover the underlying cause. Psychotherapy is indicated for patients with identifiable emotional conflicts who are sufficiently introspective to resolve anxiety of which they are consciously unaware but is being expressed as bad dreams. Patients who are unable or unwilling to look inside themselves may benefit from stress reduction techniques such as hypnosis, biofeedback, and progressive relaxation. The latter technique teaches the patient to relax an increasing number of separate muscle groups until he is completely relaxed. Administration of diazepam may suppress bad dreams if psychotherapy and/or stress reduction are ineffective; benzodiazepine should not be prescribed long-term for this purpose.

REFERENCES

Kales JD, Cadreux RJ, Saldatos CR, Kales A. Psychotherapy with night-terror patients. Amer J Psychother 1982; 36:399–407.

Kramer M. Dream disturbances. Psychiatric Ann 1979; 9:50–58.

Marshall JR. The treatment of night-terrors associated with the post-traumatic stress syndrome. Amer J Psychiatry 1975; 132:293–295.

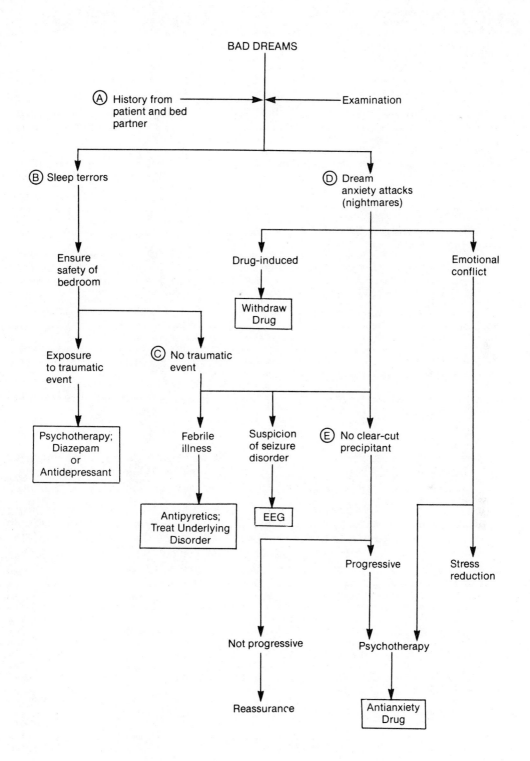

BAD DREAMS

Ⓐ History from patient and bed partner → ← Examination

Ⓑ Sleep terrors

Ⓓ Dream anxiety attacks (nightmares)

Ensure safety of bedroom

Drug-induced

Emotional conflict

Withdraw Drug

Exposure to traumatic event

Ⓒ No traumatic event

Psychotherapy; Diazepam or Antidepressant

Febrile illness

Suspicion of seizure disorder

Ⓔ No clear-cut precipitant

Antipyretics; Treat Underlying Disorder

EEG

Progressive

Stress reduction

Not progressive

Psychotherapy

Reassurance

Antianxiety Drug

SLEEP-RELATED DYSFUNCTIONS

Eric Haddes, Ph.D.

COMMENTS

A. A number of problems that do not disturb sleep and are not associated with dreams occur during the deeper levels of nonREM sleep. The patient may be less aware of the problem than a bed partner or other observer.

B. Twelve to 25 percent of children under the age of 12 experience enuresis at some time. If the patient has never been continent at night for at least 6 months, he or she is likely to have a urological abnormality.

C. Reassurance about the high rate of remission of enuresis in children, spontaneously or with any form of treatment, is appropriate when enuresis has not always been present.

D. Decreasing fluid intake while asking the child to refrain from voiding as long as possible successfully enlarges bladder capacity in one-third of patients. If enuresis is a response to a stress such as the birth of a sibling, the child's feelings about the event should be discussed. If psychotherapy is unsuccessful or no conflicts or stress are apparent, a dose of 25 mg to a maximum of 2.5 mg/kg/day of imipramine given 2 hours before bedtime usually reduces the frequency of bedwetting.

E. Enuresis in teenagers and adults is usually symptomatic of another condition, often epilepsy. Additional evidence of nocturnal seizures such as head banging or tongue biting increases the likelihood that a seizure disorder is present.

F. Patients who injure themselves while sleepwalking or have other signs of nocturnal seizures should be evaluated for epilepsy.

G. If sleepwalking has not been progressive, it is likely to be self-limited.

H. If symptoms worsen, subjects who can be hypnotized can be given the suggestion that they will waken as soon as their feet touch the floor, or simply that their sleepwalking will resolve. Diazepam may inhibit slow-wave sleep sufficiently to decrease the frequency of sleepwalking.

I. Grinding of teeth during sleep may be due to a seizure disorder if it is associated with other evidence of nocturnal seizures such as tongue biting or headbanging, or with other sleep-related disorders such as sleepwalking. Bruxism is exacerbated by alcohol consumption. In massed practice, the patient is instructed to clench and then relax his jaw for 5 seconds at a time 6 times per day for 2 weeks. Biofeedback and progressive relaxation may be useful if massed practice is unsuccessful.

REFERENCES

Lennert JB, Mowad JJ. Enuresis: evaluation of a perplexing symptom. Urology 1979; 13:27–29.

Kales A, Paulson MJ, Jacobson A, Kales J. Somnambulism: psychophysiological correlates. Arch Gen Psychiatry 1966; 11:586–604.

Arieti S, Brodie HKH, eds. American Handbook of Psychiatry. 2nd ed. New York: Basic Books, 1981: 423–454.

Ayer WA. Massed practice exercises for the elimination of tooth-grinding habits. Behav Res Ther 1976; 14:163–164.

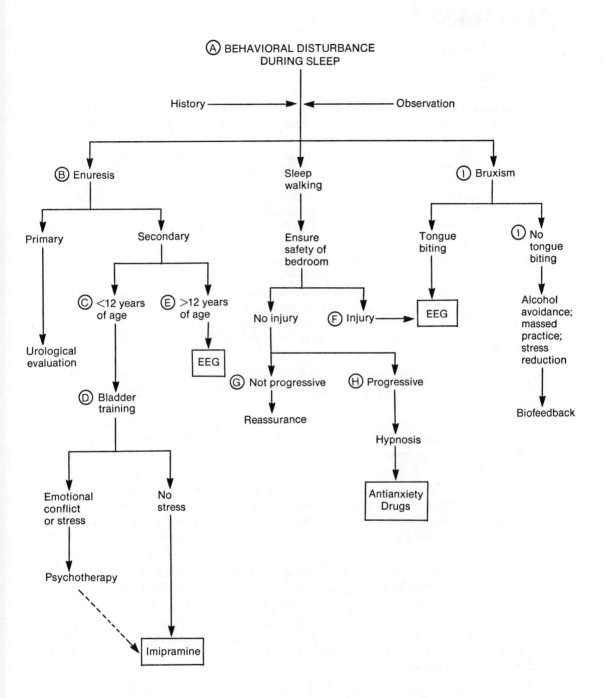

INSOMNIA

Eric Haddes, Ph.D.

COMMENTS

A. Complaints of insomnia are common (up to 75% of people); insomnia is chronic in one-third of cases. Most patients overestimate the amount of sleep deprivation, so history of the severity of insomnia from the patient alone is unreliable. The history should include: whether the patient has difficulty falling asleep, staying asleep, or wakes up early; whether insomnia occurs only in certain settings; activities, food and alcohol intake prior to bedtime; use of medications, especially sleeping preparations; pulmonary, cardiovascular, gastrointestinal, and musculoskeletal disorders that may interfere with sleep; current stresses; and changes in work schedule. The bedpartner should be asked whether the patient snores, pauses in breathing, is restless, twitches, or wakens frequently, and whether there are any problems in the relationship.

B. Depressed patients often complain of difficulty staying asleep, early morning awakening, restlessness, and fatigue. Bedtime rituals may prevent obsessive-compulsives from falling asleep. Other psychiatric disorders that may be associated with insomnia include anxiety states, phobias, psychosis, hypochondriasis, personality disorders, and organic brain syndromes. Chronic pain, alveolar hypoventilation, and gastroesophageal reflux may disrupt sleep. Insomnia in children may be due to physical discomfort, for example, from stomach aches or teething.

C. Good sleep hygiene involves using bed only for sleeping and sexual activity, regular times for sleeping and rising, avoiding daytime naps, and getting out of bed for 30 minutes if wakeful after 30 minutes.

D. If the patient's daytime wakefulness, mood, or performance are not impaired, sleep deprivation is not likely to be significant; further workup is not indicated. Biofeedback, hypnosis, meditation, breathing exercises, and progressive relaxation (pp 86–87) may help the patient fall asleep.

E. Sleeping pills and tranquilizers are ineffective for long-term use. Chronic users of these medications tend to develop difficulty staying asleep during the second half of the night. (When sedating medications are withdrawn, the dosage should be halved weekly to prevent total disruption of sleep.) Stimulants, including caffeine, taken late in the day often cause insomnia.

F. Alcoholism is associated with sleep interruptions; acute alcohol withdrawal causes increased sleep latency. A small dose of alcohol at bedtime may decrease sleep latency but is likely to disrupt sleep later at night when blood levels begin to fall.

G. Temporary sleep disturbances are common with stressful situations or with emotional excitement. Short-term administration of hypnotics at these times may prevent an acute sleep disruption from becoming chronic. Benzodiazepine hypnotics (pp 94–95) are safest and least disruptive of normal sleep.

H. When sleeping and waking times must be changed, 7-10 days may be necessary for biological rhythms to become reset. Avoidance of naps, rapid accomodation to new schedules, and blackout curtains during the day facilitate this process.

I. Nocturnal myoclonus consists of stereotyped twitching of the legs every 20–40 seconds that wakes the patient, in contrast to "hyponic jerks", which are associated with startling at sleep onset. Bedtime administration of clonozepam is the preferred treatment; other effective drugs are baclofen, carbamezapine, valproic acid, and L-trytophan when limb jerks accompany sleep apnea. Restless leg syndrome produces uncomfortable sensations in the feet and thighs while the patient is awake. When not caused by anemia, it is treated with Triavil or Percodan.

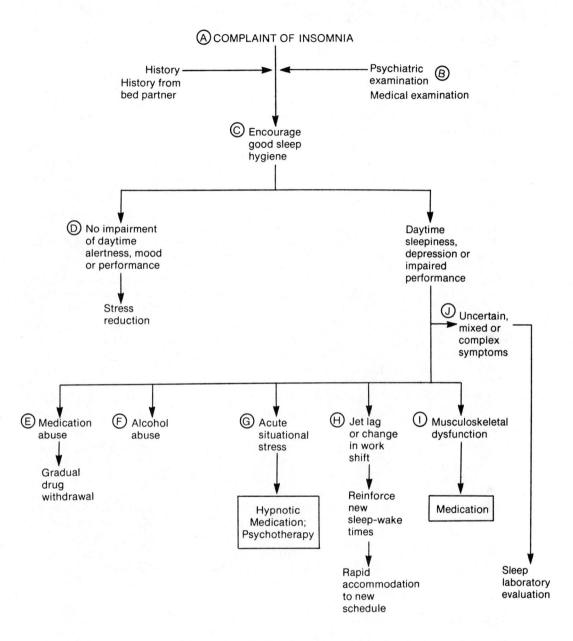

A) COMPLAINT OF INSOMNIA

History ——————→ ←—————— Psychiatric
History from   examination B)
bed partner   Medical examination

C) Encourage
good sleep
hygiene

D) No impairment
of daytime
alertness, mood
or performance

Stress
reduction

Daytime
sleepiness,
depression or
impaired
performance

J) Uncertain,
mixed or
complex
symptoms

E) Medication
abuse

F) Alcohol
abuse

G) Acute
situational
stress

H) Jet lag
or change
in work
shift

I) Musculoskeletal
dysfunction

Gradual
drug
withdrawal

Hypnotic
Medication;
Psychotherapy

Reinforce
new
sleep-wake
times

Medication

Rapid
accommodation
to new
schedule

Sleep
laboratory
evaluation

J. Diagnosis and treatment of complex conditions such as delayed and advanced sleep phase
    syndromes, require sleep laboratory testing in which the patient is observed during sleep and
    EEG, eye movements, and muscular activity are monitored.*

---

*A list of sleep disorder centers can be obtained from the Sleep Disorder Center, Stanford University Medical
School, Stanford, CA 94305 or the American Narcolepsy Association, P. O. Box 5846, Stanford, CA 94305.

REFERENCES

Guilleminault CG, Dement WC, eds. Sleep Apnea Syndromes. New York: Alan Liss, 1978.
Weitzman ED, Czeisler CA, Coleman RM, et al. Delayed sleep phase syndrome—a chronobiological
     disorder with sleep onset insomnia. Arch Gen Psychiatry 1981; 38–45.
Anon. Diagnostic Classification of Sleep and Arousal Disorders. Sleep, 1979; 2(1).
Herson M. Progress in Behavior Modification. New York: Academic Press, 1978.

EXCESSIVE DAYTIME SLEEPINESS

Eric Haddes, Ph.D.

COMMENTS

A. Use of sedating medications, nonprescription drugs, or alcohol is a frequent cause of drowsiness. Hypothyroidism, diabetes mellitus, hypoglycemia, delirium, hypothalmic disease, seizure disorders, congestive heart failure, COPD, any febrile or debilitating illness, isolation, prolonged bed rest, and boredom may produce daytime sleepiness. Women who complain of drowsiness during menstruation that is not caused by analgesics may benefit from oral contraceptives. Fatigue and sleepiness are common in the early stages of depression; emotional withdrawal may mimic drowsiness.

B. Most patients who do not sleep enough at night become drowsy during the day. If the patient has insomnia, guidelines on pp 90–91 should be followed. Even if the patient does not complain of insomnia, time spent asleep is probably inadequate if he is consistently drowsy during the day and he should be advised to increase the amount of sleep time.

C. Sleep apnea consists of multiple episodes of central and/or obstructive apnea. Snoring, restlessness, grunting, gasping, and frequent arousals suggest airway obstruction and possible hypoxemia. Obesity, hypertension and depression may be associated with obstructive sleep apnea. Sleep apnea can only be diagnosed in a sleep laboratory (pp 90–91). Hypoxemia or hypercarbia caused by pulmonary disease also may produce drowsiness. Weight reduction in obese patients with sleep apnea or poor pulmonary status may improve ventilation during sleep. Proptriptyline or medroxy progesterone for men with serious arrhythmias, improves some cases of sleep apnea. If these are ineffective, surgical correction of anatomical abnormalities that obstruct the airway during sleep may be necessary. Tracheostomy may be necessary when these measures fail to correct sleep apnea that causes significant hypertension or psychological deterioration.

D. The primary symptom of narcolepsy is the sudden onset of sleep, often at times of intense emotion. Sleep attacks may be associated with such auxiliary symptoms as sleep paralysis (paralysis of all but respiratory muscles during sleep), hypnagogic (upon falling asleep or awakening) hallucinations, cataplexy (sudden loss of motor tone while awake), and automatic behaviors. Regular daytime naps and good sleep hygiene may minimize sleep attacks. Stimulants such as pemoline, dextroamphetamine, and methylphenidate prevent sleep attacks, but they eventually lose their effectiveness. Periodic "drug holidays" decrease tolerance so that the original dose is again effective. Auxiliary symptoms of narcolepsy may be diminished by tricyclic antidepressants or monoamine oxidase inhibitors.

REFERENCES

Guilleminault C. Sleeping and Waking Disorders—Indications and Techniques. Palo Alto: Addison-Wesley, 1982.

Guilleminault C, Dement WC. 235 cases of excessive daytime sleepiness. J Neurol Sci 1977; 31:13–27.

Guilleminault C, Dement WC, Passouant P, eds. Narcolepsy. New York: Spectrum Publishing Co, 1976.

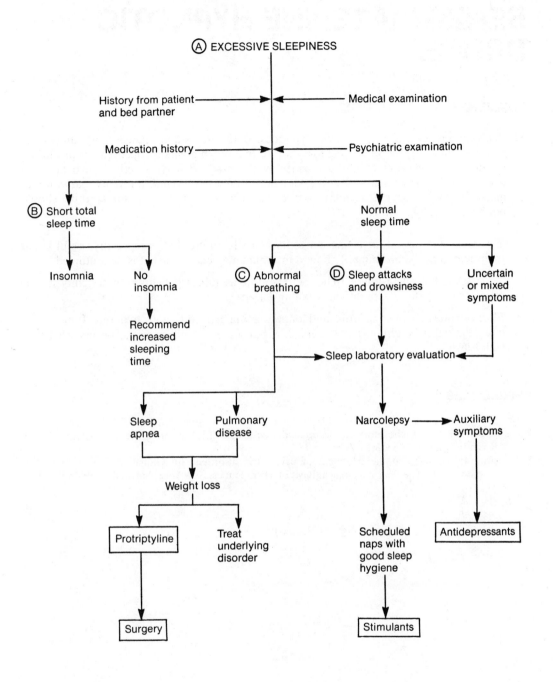

BENZODIAZEPINE HYPNOTIC DRUGS

Eric Haddes, Ph.D.

COMMENTS

A. Benzodiazepines are safe, effective hypnotics. Barbiturates and related compounds (e.g., pentobarbital, secobarbital, ethchlorvynol) have a much greater propensity for producing tolerance and life-threatening abstinence syndromes and may be lethal when taken in overdose. Unless a patient has been taking one of these compounds for many years without increasing the dose and is unwilling to discontinue it, barbiturates, and similar drugs should not be used as hypnotics.

B. Triazolam is a new short-acting benzodiazepine hypnotic that is especially useful in the treatment of initial insomnia. Rebound insomnia may occur when it is discontinued.

C. Temazepam has a half-life of 10 hours. It is more useful for patients with difficulty staying asleep than for those with difficulty falling asleep.

D. Flurazepam is the most sedating and longest-acting benzodiazepine hypnotic. It may accumulate when it is administered every day, but less rebound insomnia occurs when it is withdrawn.

REFERENCES

Kales A, Kales J. Sleep laboratory studies of hypnotic drugs: efficacy and withdrawal effects. J Clin Psychopharmacol 1983; 3:140–150.
Baldessarini RJ. Drugs and the treatment of psychiatric disorders. In: Gilman AG, Goodman LS, Gilman A, eds. The Pharmacological Basis of Therapeutics. New York: Macmillan, 1980: 391–447.

Ⓐ BENZODIAZEPINE HYPNOTIC DRUGS

Drug	Usual H.S. dosage	Half–life
Ⓑ Triazolam (Halcion)	0.25 – 0.50 mg	short
Ⓒ Temazepam (Restoril)	15 – 30 mg	intermediate
Ⓓ Flurazepam (Dalmane)	15 – 30 mg	long

ACUTE ORGANIC BRAIN SYNDROMES

Joyce S. Kobayashi, M.D.

COMMENTS

A. Between 5 and 10 percent of patients on medical and surgical wards develop acute organic brain syndromes (delirium) that may be misdiagnosed as a functional disorder, usually depression or schizophrenia. Rapid onset of symptoms in a patient without a psychiatric history suggests delirium. Predisposing factors include greater age, substance abuse, brain damage, sleep deprivation, psychological stress, sensory deprivation or overload, immobilization, and medication. The risk is highest with all centrally acting drugs, digitalis, opioids, corticosteroids, salicylates, antibiotics, antiarrhythmics, antihypertensives, antineoplastics, cimetidine, disulfiram, indomethacin and anticholinergic substances, including antidepressants, neuroleptics and over-the-counter sleeping and cold preparations. When delirium is suspected, all nonessential medications should be discontinued or the dosage reduced. Psychotropic medications should not be administered routinely to patients who may be delirious.

B. All patients experiencing an unexplained change in thinking, affect, or behavior should have a thorough mental status examination. Mental status abnormalities may only be apparent after repeated examinations because of the fluctuation characteristic of delirium. The examiner should test for fluctuating level of awareness, disorientation to time and place but not person, decreased attention, loss of short-term memory, shallow, labile affect, concrete thinking, and incoherence. Illusions, hallucinations, and delusions, are common. Delirium is usually due to diffuse cerebral dysfunction; thus, focal signs are often absent. Motor perseveration, difficulty in copying (constructional apraxia) or drawing (ideomotor apraxia) on command, and aphasia may be present. If the mental status examination is equivocal, the EEG may demonstrate slowing of the dominant rhythm or neuropsychological testing may reveal a cognitive disturbance.

C. Orientation, correction of memory deficits and a familiar environment decrease anxiety resulting from disorientation and memory loss.

D. In the absence of an abstinence syndrome, focal neurological findings should be further evaluated by CT scan.

E. CNS infections must be excluded in delirious, febrile patients who are not withdrawing from barbiturates or alcohol.

F. Seizure disorders should be considered in patients who experienced loss or alteration of consciousness prior to becoming confused.

G. Next to the effects of the illness for which the patient is being treated and the side effects of prescribed medications, intoxication with and withdrawal from alcohol and drugs are the most common causes of delirium. Blood and urine screens for psychoactive drugs are negative if delirium is caused by an abstinence syndrome. A positive barbiturate tolerance test (pp 106–107) indicates that withdrawal from tranquilizers, sleeping pills and/or alcohol are probably producing delirium. Phenobarbital or pentobarbital substituted for the offending drug must be discontinued gradually to suppress delirium and prevent seizures and hypotension.

H. Additional common causes of delirium include endocrinopathies (especially hypoglycemia and thyroid dysfunction), anemias, infections, head trauma, tumors, organ failure, seizure disorders, acid-base disturbances, and hypoxemia.

I. Any illness or poisoning that can affect the brain may cause delirium. When the mental status

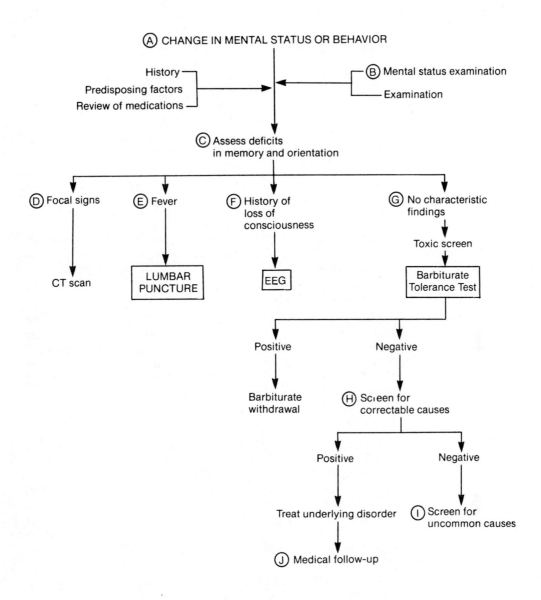

(A) CHANGE IN MENTAL STATUS OR BEHAVIOR

History ─┐
Predisposing factors
Review of medications ─┘

┌─ (B) Mental status examination
└── Examination

(C) Assess deficits in memory and orientation

(D) Focal signs

(E) Fever

(F) History of loss of consciousness

(G) No characteristic findings

Toxic screen

CT scan

LUMBAR PUNCTURE

EEG

Barbiturate Tolerance Test

Positive

Negative

Barbiturate withdrawal

(H) Screen for correctable causes

Positive

Negative

Treat underlying disorder

(I) Screen for uncommon causes

(J) Medical follow-up

examination suggests delirium, a search for an organic cause should not be abandoned even when no etiology is obvious.

J. The mortality rate immediately and at one year is higher than normal in delirious patients, even if they recover completely from the acute episode.

REFERENCES

Lipowski ZJ. Delirium: Acute Brain Failure in Man. Springfield, Illinois: CC Thomas, 1980.

Lipowski ZJ. Transient cognitive disorders in the elderly. Amer J Psychiatry 1983; 140:1426–1433.

Rabins PU, Folstein MF. Delirium and dementia: diagnostic criteria and fatality rates. Br J Psychiatry 1982; 140:149–153.

Strub RL, Black FW. Organic Brain Syndrome: An Introduction to Neurobehavioral Disorders. Philadelphia: FA Davis, 1981.

DEMENTIA

Michael G. Moran, M.D. and Troy L. Thompson II, M.D.

COMMENTS

A. In contrast to delirium, dementia is a chronic, often progressive, state of impaired mental functioning without clouded or fluctuating consciousness. Typical signs and symptoms include memory loss, personality change, depression, and loss of social skills. Focal neurological signs, paucity of gait, myoclonus, and seizures are usually absent in diffuse disease of the cerebral hemispheres until late in the course.

B. The course of the patient's illness, history indicating possible reversible causes, and the family's reaction should be ascertained. The family should be told what to expect and offered ongoing help with problem solving and grieving.

C. Reversible medical causes of dementia include abuse of CNS depressants, vitamin B12 deficiency, thyroid disease, electrolyte and mineral disturbances, normal pressure hydrocephalus, brain tumor, subdural hematoma, CNS infections, anemia, congestive heart failure, and hypoxemia. CT scan may reveal dilated ventricles or intracranial lesions; an abnormal EEG is less likely than with delirium.

D. Slow thinking, poor memory, and psychosocial deterioration caused by depression can be extremely difficult to differentiate from dementia, especially in the elderly. Depression may be present if mental status findings are inconsistent or improve with encouragement, if vegetative signs are present, if the patient complains of a cognitive deficit, or if there is a past or family history of depression. A trial of an antidepressant may be warranted even if dementia seems to be the only problem. Antidepressants tend to improve memory defects due to depression and to worsen cognitive defects caused by dementia. Lower doses may be necessary in the elderly.

E. Confusion and disorientation are decreased by familiar environment and regular reminders regarding time, place, and names. Changes should be minimized. The demented patient's ability to abstract and remember is limited; all discussions should be simple, concrete, and repetitive. Hydergine, a mixture of ergot mesyloids which is administered ($\leq$6 mg/day) in an attempt to improve cerebral blood flow, may improve depression and self-care. Lecithin (3 tbsp/day) is said to increase brain levels of acetycholine; it does not definitely improve dementia. Recent experimental attempts to increase brain levels of neurotransmitters thought to be disrupted in Alzheimer's disease have utilized IV physostigmine and intranasal desmopressin (DDAVP). Results have not yet supported the use of any definite treatment.

F. The patient whose cognition is not too disrupted can be helped to mourn the loss of previous abilities and make the most of remaining capacities. The patient should be encouraged to maintain physical and mental activity.

G. Agitation may result from anxiety and increased confusion due to worsening of brain function or changes in the environment. Even subtle physiologic derangements can result in delirium (pp 96–97) being superimposed on dementia. Common causes of delirium in this population include all prescription medications, nonprescription drugs, fever, infections, electrolyte disturbances, hypoxemia, and head injury. If orienting measures fail to decrease agitation and assaultiveness (pp 14–15) until the underlying acute disorder is corrected, haloperidol (0.5 mg–5mg/day) or propranolol (40–320 mg/day) may help.

H. It may be difficult for the family to admit the need for placing the patient outside the home. When the patient cannot be cured, the physician's ongoing involvement and willingness to try new treatments become an important source of hope that sustains the patient and his loved ones, whether or not the patient remains in the home.

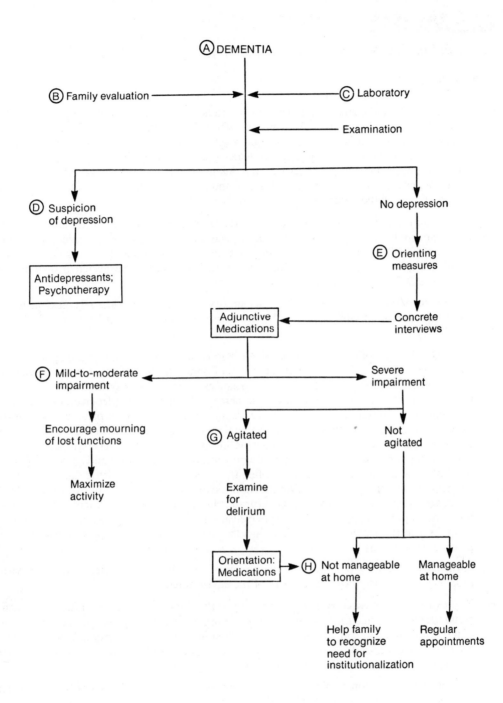

REFERENCES

Schneck MD, Riesberg B, Ferris SH. An overview of current concepts of Alzheimer's disease. Amer J
    Psychiatry 1982; 139:165–172.
Rabins PU. Reversible dementia and the misdiagnosis of dementia: a review. Hosp Comm Psychiatry 1983;
    34:830–835.
Lipowski ZJ. A new look at organic brain syndromes. Amer J Psychiatry 1980; 137:674–678.

MEMORY LOSS

Michael G. Moran, M.D. and Troy L. Thompson, II, M.D.

COMMENTS

A. Memory loss that appears in response to an obvious stress, mimics symptoms experienced by someone familiar to the patient, improves when the patient thinks that he is not being observed, or results in obvious gain may be psychogenic. A history of psychogenic memory loss, conversion symptoms, fugue, multiple personality, or conscious simulation of psychological or physical symptoms increases the likelihood that the current symptoms are functional. Whenever possible, the past history and history of the present illness should be corroborated by other sources.

B. Intoxication may produce blackouts; benzodiazepines may produce anterograde memory loss. Thorough mental status and neurological examinations are indicated. EEG may demonstrate diffuse slowing in delirium; CT scan may be useful in diagnosing dementia. A blood screen for psychoactive substances may reveal previously unsuspected drug or medication use.

C. Loss of recent memory with intact remote memory, especially with clouded consciousness or symptoms that fluctuate unpredictably or worsen at night, is characteristic of delirium (pp 96–97).

D. Before other psychotic symptoms become obvious, schizophrenic and manic patients may complain of memory problems that actually represent difficulty in concentrating. *Dissociative* disorders are acute psychogenic disturbances of memory (psychogenic amnesia and fugue), identity (multiple personality), or perception of the self (depersonalization) that represent an unconscious attempt to solve an emotional conflict by repressing awareness of the conflict along with other aspects of mental experience. The patient may not remember who he is, but he is usually able to conduct his life appropriately and may have several jobs or marriages. Functional memory difficulties may improve temporarily and a history of recent psychological stress can be obtained, when the patient is sedated with a short-acting anti-anxiety drug or is hypnotized. On the other hand, symptoms of organic brain disease tend to be worsened by any CNS depressant. Barbiturates should be avoided in patients with increased intracranial pressure, porphyria, or hypersensitivity to the drug. Treatment of psychogenic memory disturbances usually requires elucidation of stresses that are precipitating memory problems and expert psychotherapy.

E. Particularly in elderly patients, complaints of memory loss often reflect hearing or visual problems that interfere with awareness of the environment.

F. Depression may cause considerable difficulty with memory and concentration (depressive pseudodementia) which may be difficult to distinguish from true dementia. A therapeutic trial of antidepressants in patients with newly diagnosed dementia may help to distinguish between dementia and depression. Further deterioration of memory or cognition with antidepressants suggests an organic problem.

G. Patients who consciously simulate psychiatric symptoms in order to become a patient (factitious disorder) may present acutely but usually have a long history of hospitalizations under different names for improbable symptoms. Malingerers simulate memory loss to escape punishment or gain reward and usually have an underlying antisocial personality disorder (pp 138–139). Confrontation and refusal to provide inappropriate treatment should be gradual and empathic for the patient with a factitious disorder in order to increase compliance while confrontation should be immediate and firm for the malingerer.

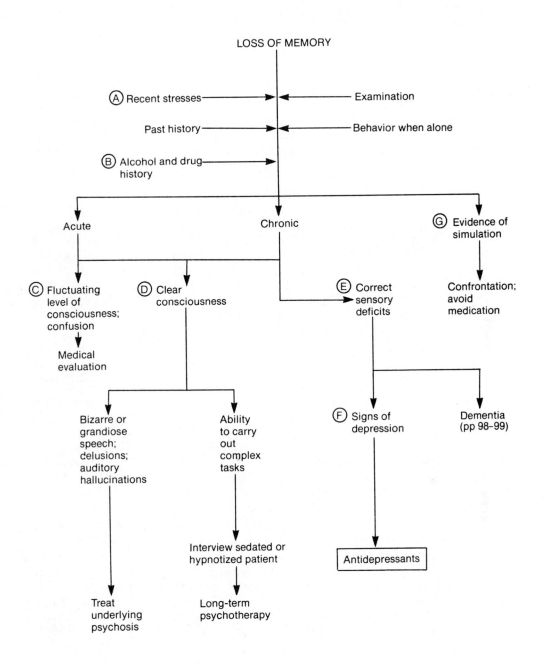

LOSS OF MEMORY

(A) Recent stresses ──────→ ←────── Examination

Past history ──────→ ←────── Behavior when alone

(B) Alcohol and drug ──────→
history

Acute

Chronic

(G) Evidence of
simulation

(C) Fluctuating
level of
consciousness;
confusion

(D) Clear
consciousness

(E) Correct
sensory
deficits

Confrontation;
avoid
medication

Medical
evaluation

Bizarre or
grandiose
speech;
delusions;
auditory
hallucinations

Ability
to carry
out
complex
tasks

(F) Signs of
depression

Dementia
(pp 98–99)

Interview sedated or
hypnotized patient

Antidepressants

Treat
underlying
psychosis

Long-term
psychotherapy

REFERENCES

Hackett TP, Cassem NH, eds. Massachusetts General Hospital Handbook of General Hospital Psychiatry. St. Louis: CV Mosby, 1978: 93–116.

Lipowski ZJ. Transient cognitive disorders (delirium, acute confusional states) in the elderly. Amer J Psychiatry 1983; 140:1426–1436.

Wells CE. Pseudodementia. Amer J Psychiatry 1979; 136:895–900.

ALCOHOLISM

Stephen L. Dilts, M.D., Ph.D.

COMMENTS

A. Indications of alcoholism include inability to carry out daily tasks without a drink, drinking in the morning, daily drinking, blackouts, impairment of physical, social, or occupational function, abstinence syndromes, binge drinking, and legal problems due to drinking. Suspicion may first be aroused by physical complications such as liver and gastrointestinal disease.

B. Family members may be important sources of information. They may also be found to be encouraging the patient to continue drinking.

C. Hospitalization is indicated for elevated vital signs (P>120, T>38.5, BP>200/90), GI bleeding, liver disease, delirium tremens, organic brain syndrome, suicide risk, psychosis, and concomitant abuse of other drugs. Hospital detoxification includes tapering doses of minor tranquilizers (e.g., diazepam 40 mg or cholorazeptate 60 mg on the first day, 30 mg on the second day, 15 mg on the third day, discontinue on the fourth day); hydration; thiamine 100 mg bid for 2 days; treatment of complications; and counseling about outpatient follow-up. Detoxification in a residential setting or at home provides consistent sleep, meals, activities, and support for abstinence without medications.

D. The major obstacles to involvement in treatment are the patient's denial of the problem and his wish to continue drinking. Denial can only be dealt with by repeated emphatic statements that the patient does have a drinking problem which is out of his control. Several such confrontations may be required.

E. The patient who is willing to consider a 1-month trial period of abstinence can usually be motivated to stop drinking; the patient who insists on any amount of continued drinking is unlikely to be able to control his alcohol intake. It is not possible to identify in advance the few patients who may be able to achieve controlled drinking; abstinence, supported by disulfiram (500 mg/day for 5 days, then 250 mg at bedtime for at least 6 months) should be the goal for most alcoholics. Contraindications to disulfiram use are organic brain syndromes or other conditions that might interfere with the patient's ability to take medication as prescribed.

F. Seventy-five percent of alcoholics have no other psychiatric disorder. A clear-cut history of psychiatric symptoms preceding onset of drinking suggests a primary psychiatric disorder. Otherwise, a period of abstinence is necessary to clarify whether alcoholism represents an attempt at self-treatment or whether psychiatric symptoms are the result of alcohol abuse. Two to four weeks of residential treatment is indicated for patients with absent or unsupportive family and friends, inadequate housing or finances, poor impulse control, inability to tolerate emotions without acting on them, and inability to be introspective. Family members should be involved in treatment efforts when possible and themselves evaluated for alcoholism.

G. All treatment approaches result in a 33% chance of significant improvement followed by relapse under stress and a 33% chance of cure. However, different approaches are compatible with different patients. Counseling programs provide advice and peer support, psychotherapy is useful to patients who see their problem as the result of psychological conflicts, Alcoholics Anonymous is appealing to those who prefer a spiritual community, and behavior therapy is most helpful to individuals who feel that alcoholism is a bad habit. Many patients benefit from a combination of approaches.

H. A crisis may make the patient realize the seriousness of his problem. Despite the frustration that results from repeated refusals of assistance, the physician must be available when the patient finally decides to ask for help.

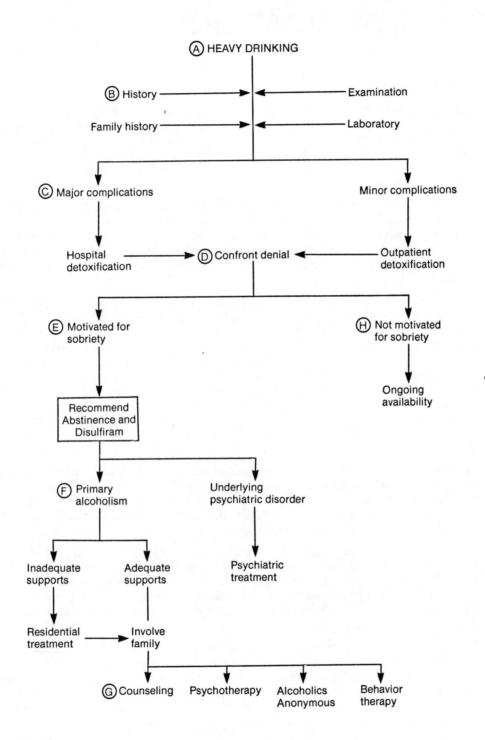

Ⓐ HEAVY DRINKING

Ⓑ History ———→ ←——— Examination

Family history ———→ ←——— Laboratory

Ⓒ Major complications   Minor complications

Hospital detoxification ———→ Ⓓ Confront denial ←——— Outpatient detoxification

Ⓔ Motivated for sobriety   Ⓗ Not motivated for sobriety

                                                    Ongoing availability

Recommend Abstinence and Disulfiram

Ⓕ Primary alcoholism   Underlying psychiatric disorder

Inadequate supports   Adequate supports   Psychiatric treatment

Residential treatment ———→ Involve family

Ⓖ Counseling   Psychotherapy   Alcoholics Anonymous   Behavior therapy

REFERENCES

Whitfield CL, Thompson G. Detoxification of 1024 alcoholic patients without psychoactive drugs. JAMA 1978; 239:1409–1410.

Gross MM, ed. Alcohol Intoxication and Withdrawal. New York: Plenum Press, 1977.

DRUG INTOXICATION
Steven L. Dubovsky, M.D.

COMMENTS

A. Ingestion of prescription or nonprescription drugs and alcohol is a frequent cause of acute psychiatric syndromes. Narcotics, CNS depressants, alcohol, and anticholinergic drugs produce confusion, disorientation, difficulty concentrating, and disturbance of short-term memory; stimulants, hallucinogens, and cannabis substances produce anxiety, paranoia, and psychosis in a clear sensorium. Specific features that differentiate intoxication syndromes are summarized on p 179.

B. Because the history from the patient is likely to be unreliable and because illicit preparations often contain mixtures of compounds of which the patient is unaware, information from additional sources, including family, associates, other physicians, pharmacies, and pill bottles, is essential. A toxic screen may be useful in identifying substances associated with dangerous intoxication and abstinence syndromes and drugs associated with violent behavior.

C. Generally speaking, severe narcotic intoxication can be attributed to variations in potency of illicit preparations; alcohol intoxication is purposeful; and barbiturate intoxication is due to accidental poisoning in addicts or to suicide attempts in non-addicts. When ingestion has been recent, guidelines for emergency treatment on pp 20–21 apply. Caffeine and stimulants do not reverse alcohol intoxication. Naloxone temporarily reverses CNS and respiratory depression caused by narcotics but not by other substances. Respiratory depression may recur up to 24 hours after apparent recovery from intoxication with most opioids and up to 72 hours after apparent recovery from methadone intoxication. Severe intoxication with CNS depressants is treated by supporting respiration and blood pressure, preventing heat loss, forced diuresis with maximal alkalinization of the urine, and dialysis if the intoxication is life-threatening.

D. Moderate intoxication with CNS depressants or anticholinergic drugs resolves when the substance is metabolized. Orienting measures (pp 96–97), reassurance, and restraint are indicated for agitation. Medications that may further depress the CNS must be avoided. IV physostigmine may temporarily reverse hyperpyrexia and CNS depression due to anticholinergic poisoning. It is more useful for diagnosis than for treatment.

E. CNS stimulants, especially amphetamine and cocaine, may produce a paranoid psychosis, which may be indistinguishable from schizophrenia, and cardiovascular hyperactivity. The patient may be assaultive, although unpredictable violent outbursts are less common than with PCP intoxication. Psychotic symptoms are treated with nonsedating neuroleptics. Hypertension and fever respond to phentolamine. Agitation should be treated according to the guidelines on pp 14–15.

F. In addition to symptoms produced by most hallucinogens, PCP may produce severe hyperactivity, violence, nystagmus, ataxia, analgesia, mutism, coma, and intracranial hemorrhage. Attempts to "talk the patient down" or any environmental stimulation may increase violence; the patient should be in a quiet room by himself. If the patient is too agitated to be left alone, restraint and intravenous sedation with haloperidol or diazepam are necessary. Seizures should be treated with intravenous diazepam.

G. Adverse reactions to hallucinogens are characterized by anxiety, inappropriate affect, depersonalization, and hallucinations. Symptoms abate with reassurance in a quiet setting and oral benzodiazepines when necessary.

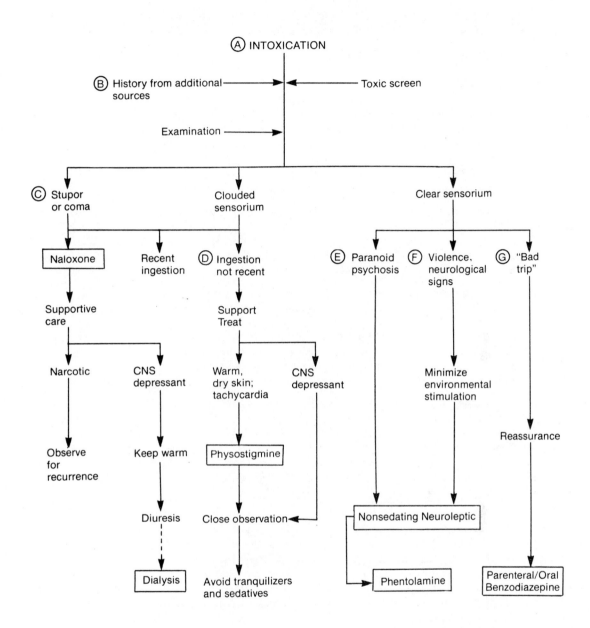

REFERENCES

Dubin WR, Stolberg R. Emergency Psychiatry for the House Officer. New York: Spectrum Publications, 1981.

Gilman AG, Goodman LS, Gilman A. The Pharmacological Basis of Therapeutics. New York: Plenum Press, 1980; 494–592.

DRUG ABSTINENCE SYNDROMES

Stephen L. Dilts, M.D., Ph.D.

COMMENTS

A. Most drugs must be administered in doses 3–4 times greater than normal for a period of at least 1 month before physical signs appear when intake is suddenly stopped; however, an abstinence syndrome may appear when long-term low-dose intake is terminated. The onset of a withdrawal syndrome may be delayed when long half-life drugs are discontinued. A history of drug use from the abusing patient alone is seldom reliable. Blood screening for psychoactive drugs may be negative, or it may reveal additional drugs.

B. Narcotic withdrawal produces lacrimation, rhinorrhea, aches and pain, abdominal cramps, chills, vomiting, diarrhea and midriasis beginning 8–12 hours after cessation of intake and lasting 7–10 days. Narcotic abstinence alone is never life-threatening. Detoxification is by substitution of methadone in a maximum dose of 20–50 mg/day and withdrawal of 10% of the total dose per day.

C. Abrupt withdrawal from amphetamines, methylphenidate, and cocaine can produce lethargy, apathy, depression, hypersomnia, nightmares, and increased appetite but is not inherently lethal unless the patient becomes suicidal. Patients with intact psychosocial supports can be withdrawn on an outpatient basis. In the absence of supports, reversion to drug use is likely; hospitalization is necessary to find alternative coping strategies. Hospitalization is also indicated for suicidal thoughts because of the high risk of impulsive behavior. Imipramine in standard doses may reverse severe depression caused by stimulant withdrawal.

D. Withdrawal from sedative-hypnotics, tranquilizers, and alcohol can result in insomnia, CNS irritability, hyperreflexia, tachycardia, fever, postural hypotension, seizures, delirium, and cardiovascular collapse. Alcohol withdrawal is treated by hydration, minor tranquilizers and thiamine (pp 102–103). Abstinence from barbiturates and related compounds can be life-threatening and requires close monitoring. The barbiturate abstinence syndrome begins 12–24 hours after drug discontinuation, peaks in about 4 days, and lasts about 7 days.

E. Barbiturates, meprobamate, ethchlorvynol, glutelhimide, methyprylon, chloral hydrate, benzodiazepines, and alcohol produce cross-tolerance. When the patient no longer appears intoxicated, 200 mg of pentobarbital or 60–100 mg of phenobarbital are administered on an empty stomach to determine the degree of tolerance to any combination of these substances. If the patient falls asleep or becomes markedly drowsy, he is not tolerant and will not experience an abstinence syndrome. Dysarthria, nystagmus, and ataxia without sleepiness indicate moderate tolerance. The patient will need 200–300 mg of pentobarbital or 60–90 mg of phenobarbital per day to suppress withdrawal symptoms. Absence of symptoms, or nystagmus only, after the test dose indicates that the patient is markedly tolerant and will need 400–500 mg of pentobarbital or 150–180 mg of phenobarbital per day. An alternative method is to administer 60–100 mg of phenobarbital every 1–4 hours until the patient becomes intoxicated. Once the dose of medication necessary to prevent withdrawal is determined, the drug is withdrawn at a rate of 10% of the total dose of phenobarbital every other day, or more rapidly with pentobarbital. If there is any possibility that a CNS depressant in addition to alcohol has been abused, a barbiturate tolerance test should be performed.

F. Close outpatient follow-up is required to monitor for a return to drug abuse following discharge from hospital.

REFERENCES

Majehrewrez E, Noble EP, eds. Biochemistry and Pharmacology of Ethanol. New York: Plenum Press, 1979.

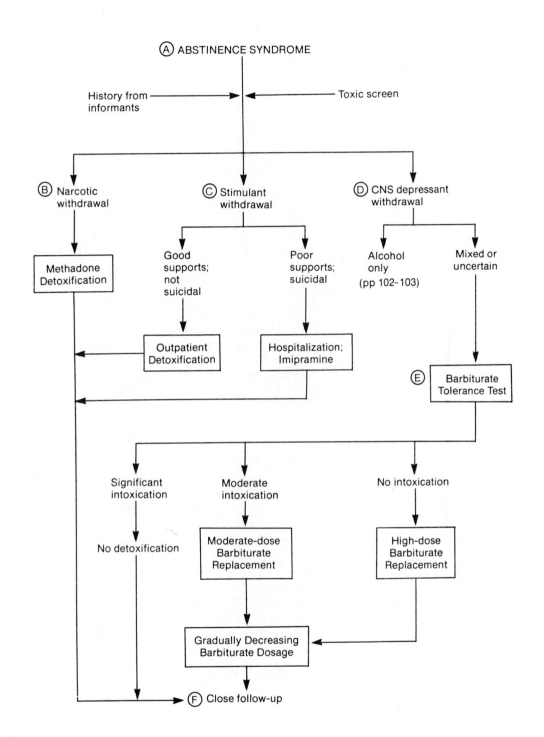

Robinson GM. Barbiturate hypno-sedative withdrawal by a multiple oral phenobarbital loading dose technique. Clin Pharmacol Ther 1981; 30:71–76.

NARCOTIC ABUSE
Stephen L. Dilts, M.D., Ph.D.

COMMENTS

A. Excepting patients who receive narcotics by prescription, abusers of opiates (e.g., heroin, morphine, hydromorphone, codeine) and related compounds (e.g., propoxyphene, pentazocine, meperidine) should eventually have drugs withdrawn. Narcotic abstinence may lead to mild influenza and other minor problems, but the main obstacle to successful withdrawal is the addict's psychological dependence which leads to continued drug-seeking behavior. Obtain from the patient, and from other observers who may be more reliable, a history of other abused drugs including alcohol. Needle tracks, suspicious complaints, "lost" prescriptions, requests for specific drugs or large amounts, and threatening behavior when narcotics are not prescribed suggest narcotic abuse.

B. Indications for ongoing narcotic administration to addicted patients include acute medical and surgical illness, terminal illness, and pregnancy. Although drug maintenance is safer for the fetus than withdrawal, abstinence in the newborn can present serious problems. Because of their tolerance, physically ill addicts require higher doses of narcotics.

C. Patients who have been abusing narcotics for more than a year find it extremely difficult to stop relying on drugs. A period of methadone maintenance is helpful in stabilizing the patient's life, solidifying a relationship with the therapist, and helping the patient to find new ways of coping with stress. Federal guidelines for maintaining addicts on methadone require administration by a federally approved physician, and evidence of tolerance such as a corroborated history of drug abuse, withdrawal symptoms, signs of drug administration (e.g., needle tracks, pinpoint pupils, nodding), and complications (e.g., endocarditis, hepatitis).

D. Strong external (e.g., stable job, adequate finances, intact family, healthy hobbies, religion) and internal (e.g., intact self-esteem, impulse control, physical health, coping abilities) supports help the patient to tolerate withdrawal of narcotics without an extended intermediate period of methadone maintenance.

E. Methadone maintenance is used to stabilize the patient's life in order to facilitate efforts to restructure internal and external psychosocial supports. Typical *maintenance* doses range from 20 to 50 mg daily, although some addicts require as much as 100 mg. Regular urinalysis is necessary to monitor ongoing drug abuse.

F. The usual starting dose for detoxification is 20 mg given once daily, increased in 5–mg steps to no more than 40–50 mg per day or until symptoms of withdrawal are suppressed, and then decreased by 5 mg per day until withdrawn. Adjunctive medications may include antianxiety drugs (e.g., chlorazepate 15 mg for one day, tapered over 3 to 4 days), hydroxyzine 25 to 50 mg every 4 to 6 hours for nausea, and clonidine 0.3–0.4 mg tapered over 2–4 weeks to decrease abstinence symptoms.

G. Some form of counseling is necessary after the patient is withdrawn to help him to adjust to a drug-free life. Recovered addicts may be extremely important members of a team that emphasizes restructuring the patient's identity and acquisition and strengthening of coping skills. Although antidepressants may be necessary during this time, potentially addicting antianxiety drugs should be avoided.

REFERENCES

Senay E. Substance Abuse Disorders in Clinical Practice. New York: John Wright Publishing, 1983.

Wikler A. Diagnosis and treatment of drug dependence of the barbiturate type. Amer J Psychiatry 1968; 125:758–765.

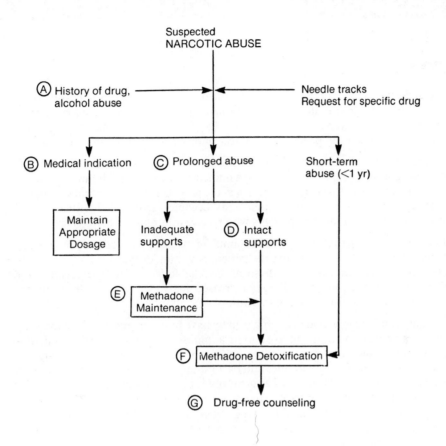

Suspected
NARCOTIC ABUSE

Ⓐ History of drug, ──────→ ←────── Needle tracks
alcohol abuse   Request for specific drug

Ⓑ Medical indication   Ⓒ Prolonged abuse   Short-term
abuse (<1 yr)

```
┌──────────────┐
│   Maintain   │        Inadequate      Ⓓ Intact
│ Appropriate  │        supports           supports
│   Dosage     │
└──────────────┘
```

Ⓔ ┌──────────────┐
│ Methadone   │ ──────→
│ Maintenance │
└──────────────┘

Ⓕ ┌─────────────────────────────┐
│   Methadone Detoxification   │ ←──────
└─────────────────────────────┘

Ⓖ   Drug-free counseling

PRESCRIBING ADDICTIVE DRUGS

Stephen L. Dilts, M.D., Ph.D.

COMMENTS

A. When the physician is unfamiliar with a patient, requests for potentially addictive drugs must be evaluated very carefully. Even in an ongoing relationship, the patient may be abusing medications without the doctor's knowledge. Some patients may describe complaints in convincing detail, even producing physical findings in order to simulate disease.

B. Adequate doses of analgesics should be prescribed for bona fide acute pain syndromes if the patient agrees to regular follow-up and a limited period of drug administration. Addicts need 2–3 times the usual doses of narcotics for acute pain. Underprescription actually increases the risk of addiction because the patient may become preoccupied with pain and its relief. Addiction is rare in medical patients who receive appropriate analgesia.

C. Factors suggesting that symptoms are simulated to obtain drugs include: unlikely or inconsistent symptoms; statement that the patient is visiting or that his physician is on vacation; absence of corroboration by a physician or reliable family member; request for a specific drug; anger, threatening behavior, or increased demands when the physician is reluctant to prescribe; signs of drug abuse, intoxication, or withdrawal.

D. Chronic pain, anxiety, and insomnia usually have both organic and functional components. Before making a commitment to ongoing administration of potentially addicting drugs, the physician should rule out reversible emotional disorders that may produce symptoms. Increasing doses of most narcotics and barbiturates often are necessary to produce the same effect; the risk of addiction is not as great but is present with benzodiazepines. Patients who cannot agree to limit long-term drug intake or who demonstrate a high potential for drug abuse should receive treatment for drug abuse (pp 108–109). Repeated confrontations and refusal to prescribe may be necessary to help the patient to see that drug-seeking behavior has become an important part of his life.

E. Patients with chronic symptoms who can agree to limited daily maintenance doses, are able to form a stable relationship with the physician, keep appointments regularly, and have viable psychosocial supports, can benefit from ongoing administration of appropriate drugs. It may be helpful to prepare an explicit, written agreement about size and duration of prescriptions, plans for tapering doses, and use of adjunctive treatment modalities such as massage, biofeedback, and hypnosis. Such treatment contracts should be reviewed at least every 6 months. The most useful medication for the long-term treatment of pain is methadone, which can be given in a once-daily dose, has little effect on mental functioning, and produces little euphoria. Long-acting benzodiazepines such as chlorazepate or diazepam are useful for chronic anxiety and insomnia; they produce fewer rebound symptoms on withdrawal and can be administered in one or two daily doses.

REFERENCES

Ewing JA. Diagnosis and management of depressant drug dependence. Amer J Psychiatry 1967; 123:909–917.

Clouet DH, ed. Narcotic Drugs: Biomechanical Pharmacology. New York: Plenum Press, 1971.

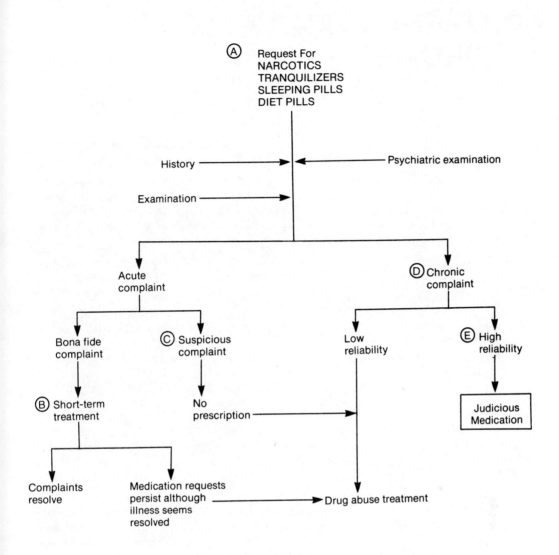

ACUTE DRUG AND ALCOHOL SYNDROMES
Steven L. Dubovsky, M.D.

COMMENTS

A. Specific manifestations of intoxication vary for different prescription and nonprescription drugs and alcohol. A general approach to management is outlined on pp 106–107.

B. This column describes substances that are commonly used as adulterants of illicit preparations of the drug and other substances that are likely to be abused at the same time. Intoxication or withdrawal may be more dangerous when these additional substances are present. Contaminants of narcotic preparations may contribute to medical complications such as abscesses, endocarditis, and septicemia.

C. Signs and symptoms are listed in the order of their appearance with greater levels of intoxication.

D. Alcohol abstinence syndromes include:
   1) Alcohol withdrawal ("the shakes"). Tremulousness, tachycardia, nausea, diaphoresis, orthostatic hypotension, and weakness appear within a few hours of decreasing or stopping alcohol consumption and last 3–7 days.
   2) Major motor seizures ("rum fits"). Seizures appear during the first 48 hours in a few cases of the shakes.
   3) Alcohol withdrawal delirium (delirium tremens or "DTs"). Delirium, autonomic hyperactivity, agitation, gross tremulousness, and hallucinations begin on the 2nd—3rd day of abstinence in patients who have been drinking heavily for 5–15 years.
   4) Alcohol hallucinosis. Threatening or derogatory auditory hallucinations with a clear sensorium appear within 48 hours of cessation of drinking, or with a decrease in intake at the end of a long binge. Symptoms last a few hours–days but persist for weeks–months in 10% of cases. Hallucinosis occasionally becomes chronic, in which case it may be indistinguishable from schizophrenia.

E. Barbiturates and related compounds include phenobarbital, amobarbital, pentobarbital, secobarbital, chloral hydrate, ethchlorvynol, glutethimide, meprobamate, methyprylon, and methaqualone (recently removed from the market). Short-acting preparations such as amobarbital are lethal at lower doses than long-acting preparations such as phenobarbital. Benzodiazepines include diazepam, oxazepam, chlordiazepoxide, lorazepam, prazepam, chlorazepate, alprazolam, flurazepam, temazepam, and triazolam.

F. Narcotics include morphine, heroin, hydromorphone, oxymorphone, levorphanol, codeine, hydrocodone, oxycodone, methadone, meperidine, alphaprodine, and propoxyphene. Pentazocine has both narcotic antagonist and agonist properties.

G. CNS stimulants include amphetamines, methylphenidate, cocaine, phenmetrazine, and phenylpropanolamine. Tolerance develops to many effects but not to the capacity to produce a toxic psychosis.

H. Hallucinogens include LSD, psilocybin, mescaline, PCP, and STP. Cannabis substances, which are much less likely to produce hallucinations, include marijuana, hashish, and THC.

I. Most over-the-counter cold and sleeping preparations are anticholinergic, as are atropine, belladonna, henbane, scopolamine, antiparkinsonian drugs, many tricyclic antidepressants, some neuroleptics, Jimson weed, mandrake, and propantheline.

REFERENCE

Bowers MB. Acute psychosis induced by psychotomimetic drug abuse. Arch Gen Psychiatry 1972; 27:437–442.

ACUTE DRUG AND ALCOHOL SYNDROMES [A]

Class	Drugs Common [B] in Mixed Abuse and Adulterants	Manifestations of Intoxication [C]	Abstinence Syndrome
CNS Depressants Alcohol	Barbiturates, minor tranquilizers	Disorganized cognitive and motor processes, overconfidence, mood swings, increased pain threshold, hypothermia, increased intra-cranial pressure, stupor, coma. Death rare in uncomplicated unconscious-ness lasting < 12 hours.	[D] Withdrawal Major seizures Delirium Hallucinosis
Barbiturates and related compounds [E]	Alcohol, benzodiazepines	Euphoria, increased pain threshold nystagmus, ataxia, dysarthria, postural hypotension, hypothermia, stupor, coma, cardiovascular collapse. Barbiturates are much more lethal than benzodiazepines.	Anxiety, agitation, CNS irritability, seizures, cardiovascular collapse. Symptoms begin within 12–24 hours, peak at 4–7 days, and last one week. Withdrawal syndrome appears later and lasts longer after discontinuation of long–acting compounds.
Benzodiazepines	Alcohol; barbiturates		
Narcotics [F]	Quinine, procaine, lidocaine, lactose, mannitol, bacteria, viruses, fungi	Analgesia, drowsiness, nausea and vomiting, lethargy, euphoria, miosis, flushed warm skin, respiratory depression, coma, shock.	Lacrimation, rhinorrhea, restlessness, sleepiness, gooseflesh, yawning, irritability, coryza. Symptoms appear 8–12 hours after drug cessation, peak at 48–72 hours, and last 7–10 days.
CNS Stimulants [G]	Barbiturates	Elevated mood, increased energy, midriasis, anorexia, irritability, insomnia, hypertension, tachycardia, fever, psychosis with paranoia, visual, auditory and tactile hallucinations, and delusions of infestation, all in a clear sensorium; intracranial hemorrhage (rare).	Increased sleep and appetite, nightmares, depression, suicide.
Hallucinogens [H]	Stimulants	Anxiety, depersonalization, distortion of time sense, dilated pupils, increased heart rate and blood pressure, paranoia, illusions, hallucinations. PCP also causes violence, coma, mutism, analgesia, nystagmus, ataxia.	None. Flashbacks may be precipitated by marijuana or antihistamines.
Cannabis substances	Stimulants	Euphoria, anxiety, suggestibility, increased appetite, distortions of time and space, injected conjunctivae, pupils unchanged.	
Anticholinergics [I]	May be contained in herbal preparations	Confusion, delirium, drowsiness, tachycardia, fever, warm dry skin, body image distortions, fixed dilated pupils.	Mania.

ERECTILE DYSFUNCTION

Daniel A. Hoffman, M.D.

COMMENTS

A. Impotence is primary if the man has never had an erection with a partner, in which case it is likely to have an organic etiology, and secondary if the patient has been potent at least one time with a partner in the past. Erections may be partial, or completely absent. A psychogenic etiology is suggested if erections occur in the morning, with masturbation, and with one partner or sexual activity but not another. Absent nocturnal penile tumescence indicates an organic cause of impotence (35% of cases). Careful general and urologic examinations and a review of medications that may cause erectile dysfunction are indicated to investigate possible physical etiologies.

B. Marital conflicts may be expressed in impotence (pp 174–175); problems in the marriage may result from incurable impotence.

C. The man may need help in dealing with anger, humiliation, loss of a valued function, and fears that his partner will abandon him if irreversible organic pathology produces permanent impotence. The couple may be helped to find alternative means of sexual fulfillment or to explore the possibility of a penile prosthesis.

D. Impotence of uncertain etiology should be treated as functional while studies such as nocturnal penile tumescence, penile Doppler studies, testosterone, prolactin, LH and FSH levels are performed. Failure of sex and couples therapy indicates a more intensive search for an organic cause and consideration of a prosthesis.

E. Fear of being unable to attain an erection or otherwise perform sexually (performance anxiety) results in the patient's attention being focused on erections rather than on other aspects of sex. When the patient becomes overly concerned about performance, anxiety increases, further decreasing sexual functioning. Performance anxiety is ameliorated by paying attention to the pleasurable aspects of physical closeness while thinking less about erection. During pleasuring sessions without genital contact, the patient is instructed to concentrate on enjoying sensual pleasure. Erections usually begin to appear spontaneously when performance anxiety is decreased and physical pleasure increased. The couple is then instructed to enjoy any erections that occur but to refrain from genital contact and continue physical pleasuring after erections recede. Multiple experiences with erections reappearing after they have receded teaches the patient and his partner not to be concerned about losing erections.

F. Once the patient has gained confidence in spontaneous erections, genital contact is gradually introduced. Initially, erections that occur are allowed to recede. Manually or orally produced orgasms are permitted, but intercourse is prohibited until confidence in the ability to sustain or regain an erection is strong. The couple then proceeds to intercourse in the female-superior position with minimal thrusting or bedding of the shaft of the penis, progressing very gradually to intercourse in other positions. Regressions, which are common, indicate a need to return to the previous stage.

REFERENCES

Masters W, Johnson V. Human Sexual Inadequacy. Boston: Little, Brown, 1970.

Kaplan HS. The New Sex Therapy. New York: Brunner/Mazel, 1974.

Kaplan HS. Disorders of Sexual Desire. New York: Brunner/Mazel, 1974.

Spark J. Impotence is not always psychogenic. JAMA 1980; 243:750–755.

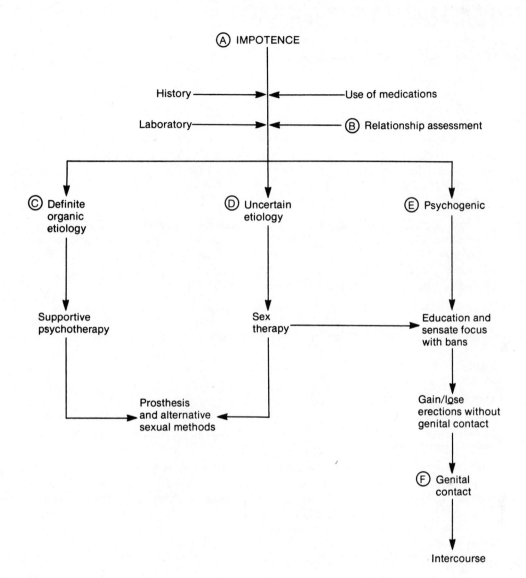

FEMALE ORGASMIC DYSFUNCTION

Daniel A. Hoffman, M.D.

COMMENTS

A. Due to the anatomical location of the clitoris, two-thirds of all women are not regularly orgasmic through intercourse without some form of direct clitoral stimulation. A number of illnesses and medications can alter libido and orgasmic function (pp 118–119), as can depression and marital conflict. Note whether the woman is orgasmic in some situations but not others.

B. Every anorgasmic woman should receive a thorough pelvic examination. If pubococcygeal muscles are lax, exercises to strengthen them may enhance clitoral stimulation during intercourse. The patient is instructed to contract the muscles by closing the urethral and anal sphincters and performing a Valsalva maneuver. Exercises should be repeated frequently, at least 6 times per day with 10 repetitions per session.

C. Women who are orgasmic with masturbation or oral sex but not intercourse are likely to be receiving inadequate clitoral stimulation during intercourse. The couple should be taught to stimulate the clitoris directly before, during, or after intercourse. Increased clitoral stimulation during intercourse may be provided by the female-superior position which permits more direct contact between the clitoris and the man's pubic symphisis, and by manual manipulation during intercourse.

D. Possibly because their primary problem is that they have not learned about their own sexual response, women who have never been orgasmic through any means including masturbation (primary orgasmic dysfunction) tend to be more likely to become regularly orgasmic than those who have been orgasmic in the past.

E. Before proceeding with partner techniques, the woman should be taught to pleasure herself in a private setting with the goal of learning about her body's sensual responses rather than experiencing orgasm. Fantasy should be encouraged using printed materials if desired, and the woman should increasingly explore her genitals. Self-help books may be useful in guiding this exploration. A vibrator may be used, but it should not be the only form of stimulation as it may become addictive.

F. Pressure to perform by experiencing an orgasm is removed by a ban on intercourse; the woman teaches her partner, verbally and by placing his hands where she wants them, those forms of manipulation that are most pleasurable to her. The focus is initially on the pleasurable aspects of sexual play and ways in which clitoral stimulation can be incorporated into lovemaking.

G. If the woman still is not orgasmic with intercourse, the couple should be taught to provide clitoral stimulation before or after intercourse. Concerns about being unable to experience orgasm through intercourse alone should be elicited and the couple reassured that this may be normal.

REFERENCES

Masters W, Johnson V. Human Sexual Inadequacy. Boston: Little, Brown, 1970.
Kaplan HS. The New Sex Therapy. New York: Brunner/Mazel, 1974.
Kaplan HS. Disorders of Sexual Desire. New York: Brunner/Mazel, 1974.
Spark J. Impotence is not always psychogenic. JAMA 1980; 243:750–755.

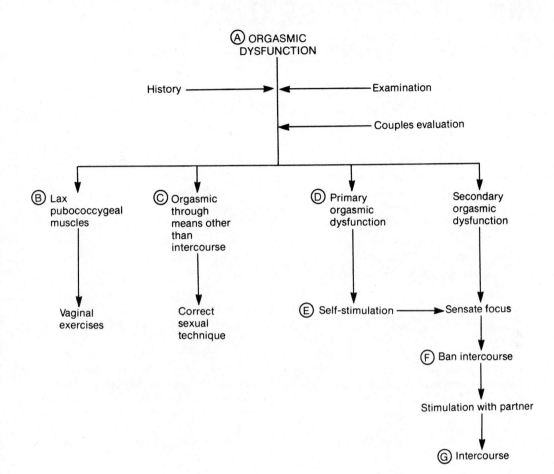

A ORGASMIC
DYSFUNCTION

History ⟶ ⟵ Examination

⟵ Couples evaluation

B Lax
pubococcygeal
muscles

C Orgasmic
through
means other
than
intercourse

D Primary
orgasmic
dysfunction

Secondary
orgasmic
dysfunction

Vaginal
exercises

Correct
sexual
technique

E Self-stimulation ⟶ Sensate focus

F Ban intercourse

Stimulation with partner

G Intercourse

APPROACH TO SEXUAL DYSFUNCTION

Daniel Hoffman, M.D.

COMMENTS

A. Because of embarrassment or uncertainty the patient with sexual dysfunction often is reluctant to discuss the problem unless the clinician indicates an interest through direct questions. *Primary* sexual problems have always been present; *secondary* problems are new. Determine whether the dysfunction is associated with alcohol or drug use, whether it occurs with all partners and with masturbation or with one partner. Routine evaluation includes a sexual history highlighting recent changes in sexual functioning and satisfaction of both partners with sex, with an interview of the couple together when possible.

B. Testosterone levels, penile Doppler studies, and occasionally, arteriography will differentiate organic from functional impotence. A vaginal smear may reveal a hormonal imbalance causing difficulty with lubrication.

C. Organic impotence is characterized by a history of no erections during dreaming and in the early morning, and 3 or more episodes of absent nocturnal penile tumescence. Illnesses that result in sexual dysfunction include: loss of libido (cerebral, ovarian, or adrenal disease, chronic illness); erectile dysfunction, loss of libido (pulmonary, renal, cardiac, liver, and endocrine disease, malignancy, Lerich syndrome, genitourinary disease); premature or retarded ejaculation (prostatitis, urethritis, lumbar sympathectomy, abdominal aortic surgery); impotence, orgasmic dysfunction (multiple sclerosis, amyotrophic lateral sclerosis, diabetes mellitus); and orgasmic dysfunction, vaginismus (dysparunia). Certain medications may affect sexual function (e.g., CNS depressants and estrogens may cause decreased libido, while anabolic agents and androgens can increase libido). Impotence may be produced by alcohol, spironolactone, guanethidine, methyldopa, tranquilizers, tricyclic antidepressants, and cimetidine.

D. When treatment of a physical disorder does not improve sexual functioning, the patient and his or her spouse can be helped to overcome loss of self-esteem and grief at relinquishing habitual approaches and find alternative means of sexual fulfillment (e.g., through foreplay or oral sex rather than intercourse, and penile prostheses for irreversible erectile dysfunction).

E. Sexual dysfunction may mask a primary psychiatric disorder in one partner such as depression, anxiety or substance abuse, or it may indicate a more significant problem in the relationship, most commonly anger, infidelity, and jealousy when a newborn child receives more attention than the husband or wife. Such problems can be uncovered by asking how each partner has felt about the relationship and about recent changes in the relationship. Even when the focus is on individual psychopathology, treatment efforts should also be directed toward the couple (conjoint therapy) to deal with the partner's reaction to the patient's behavior and to help correct pathological patterns that have developed. If sexual problems do not resolve with this approach, sex therapy should be considered. Sex therapy is most effective when both people are involved. It is important to evaluate the couple's capacity to tolerate the intimacy that is created by daily assignments requiring physical contact and open discussions.

F. When sexual problems occur in the context of an unstable relationship, conjoint therapy to resolve major difficulties should precede sex therapy to help the couple tolerate the procedure. If discussion of problems leads to dissolution of the marriage, it is likely that this outcome was inevitable.

G. Sex therapy is a time limited treatment in which the couple carries out assigned exercises 5 days per week. After a thorough sexual history is obtained, a ban is placed on intercourse.

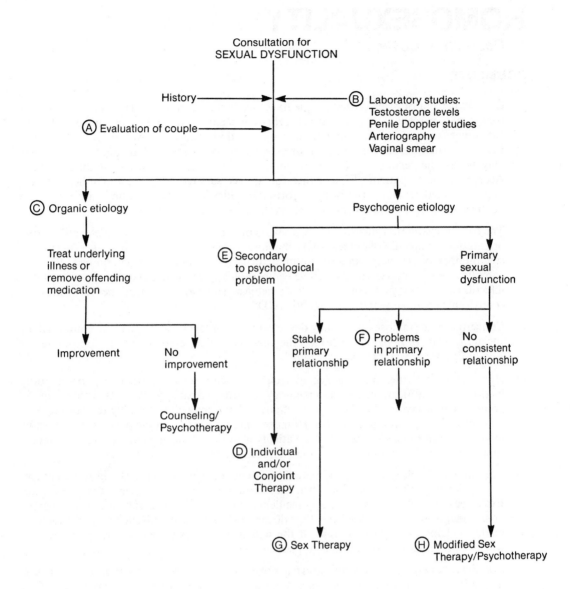

Consultation for
SEXUAL DYSFUNCTION

History

Ⓐ Evaluation of couple

Ⓑ Laboratory studies:
Testosterone levels
Penile Doppler studies
Arteriography
Vaginal smear

Ⓒ Organic etiology

Psychogenic etiology

Treat underlying
illness or
remove offending
medication

Ⓔ Secondary
to psychological
problem

Primary
sexual
dysfunction

Improvement

No
improvement

Stable
primary
relationship

Ⓕ Problems
in primary
relationship

No
consistent
relationship

Counseling/
Psychotherapy

Ⓓ Individual
and/or
Conjoint
Therapy

Ⓖ Sex Therapy

Ⓗ Modified Sex
Therapy/Psychotherapy

"Sensate focus" exercises (pp 122–123) help the couple to learn to communicate ways in which they would like to be stimulated, first without and then with genital contact. Specific techniques are then taught for dysfunctions, and intercourse is gradually reinstated.

H. Occasionally, treatment of a sexual dysfunction in an individual who does not have a regular relationship can be accomplished with group therapy, education about sexual physiology and function, and help in recognition of stresses that occur during sex. Psychotherapy should be directed toward helping the patient to find a regular partner who can then be involved in ongoing sex therapy.

HOMOSEXUALITY

Deborah A. Coyle, M.D.

COMMENTS

A. Over 50 percent of heterosexual people have engaged in transient homosexual behavior at some time; 3 percent of women and 6 percent of men have a strictly homosexual orientation. Effeminacy in men and masculine traits in women do not correlate with sexual orientation. Many homosexuals have no concerns or medical complaints related to homosexuality; they may worry that exposure of their orientation will adversely effect their medical care. Acceptance of the patient's lifestyle therefore is necessary to encourage him or her to reveal important medical and psychosocial information. Physicians who feel uncomfortable with homosexual patients should consider referral.

B. The routine evaluation should include a sexual history; begin by asking the patient's sexual orientation. Frequency of homosexual behavior, history of recent encounters, specific practices, number of partners, and concomitant drug abuse should be determined. Physical complications of homosexuality include hemorrhoids, anal fissures and sexually transmitted infections, including gonorrhea, syphillis, amebiasis, shigellosis, hepatitis, perirectal abscess, condylomata acumata, and, presumably, AIDS.

C. Concerns about homosexuality may develop in the context of some medical, emotional, or social problem, or in patients who feel they may have characteristics of the opposite sex or who have homosexual fantasies.

D. Homosexual activities may be due to lack of a heterosexual partner, experimentation, inadequate identification, feminist ideology, or true bisexuality. Patients who engage in homosexual behavior when heterosexual partners are unavailable usually revert to heterosexuality when the situation changes. Homosexual rape victims should be treated in the same manner as heterosexual rape victims. Patients with uncertain or mixed sexual preferences should be evaluated for depression and character pathology.

E. The patient who clearly has a homosexual preference may need some help adjusting. Patients may seek support and education when they are ambivalent about their sexual preference. Exclusive homosexuals have no higher incidence of psychopathology, antisocial behavior, or dissatisfaction with their sexual lives than do heterosexuals. Generally, no attempts should be made to change sexual orientation. If the patient expresses a wish to change, determine whether his principle motivation is to please others.

F. Conflicts about being homosexual and fears of discovery may result in symptoms of anxiety; the patient may attempt to suppress anxiety with forced heterosexual behavior. The Gay Coalition and similar organizations can be important sources of information and support.

G. Depression is frequently related to problems with a lover; the partner should be involved in treatment if possible (pp 174–175). Rejection by family, concerns about aging and about contracting a life-threatening disease also commonly cause depression.

H. Disorders of potency, lubrication, libido, and orgasm are treated as they would be in heterosexuals (pp 118–119).

REFERENCES

Kentsmith DK, Eaton MK. Treating Sexual Problems in Medical Practice. New York: Arco Publishing, 1979.

Lief HI, ed. Sexual Problems in Medical Practice. Chicago: American Medical Association, 1981.

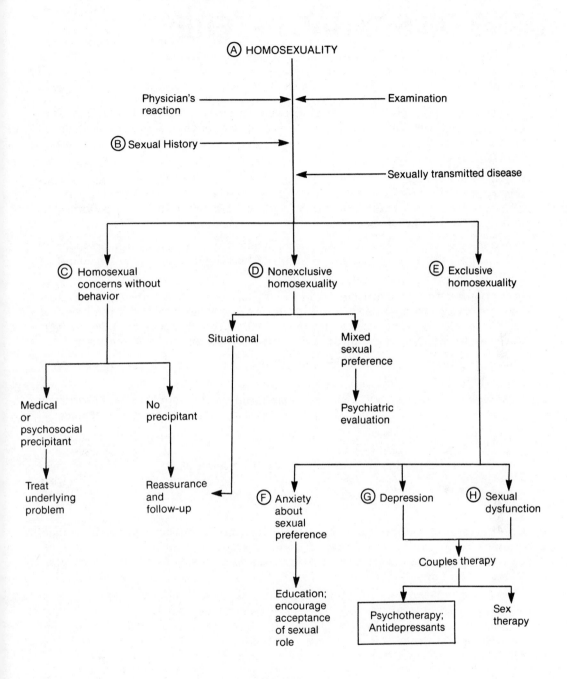

Ⓐ HOMOSEXUALITY

Physician's ──────→ ←────── Examination
reaction

Ⓑ Sexual History ──────────→

←────── Sexually transmitted disease

Ⓒ Homosexual
concerns without
behavior

Ⓓ Nonexclusive
homosexuality

Ⓔ Exclusive
homosexuality

Situational

Mixed
sexual
preference

Psychiatric
evaluation

Medical
or
psychosocial
precipitant

No
precipitant

Treat
underlying
problem

Reassurance
and
follow-up

Ⓕ Anxiety
about
sexual
preference

Ⓖ Depression

Ⓗ Sexual
dysfunction

Couples therapy

Education;
encourage
acceptance
of sexual
role

Psychotherapy;
Antidepressants

Sex
therapy

121

LOSS OF SEXUAL INTEREST

Daniel A. Hoffman, M.D.

COMMENTS

A. Disinterest in sex may result from: early experiences, problems in an important relationship, frightening, embarrassing, or traumatic sexual encounters, or physical or psychiatric illness. Since marital conflict is a frequent cause of loss of libido, both partners should be evualated (pp 174–175).

B. Chronic debilitating illnesses, pain, fatigue, disorders specifically affecting potency, genitourinary and venereal diseases may result in loss of interest in sex. Antihypertensives, coritcosteroids, tranquilizers, narcotics and alcohol also decrease sexual drive and performance, while cocaine and amphetamines may produce a transient increase.

C. Depression, anxiety, obsessions, and schizophrenia may disrupt sexual interest due to emotional withdrawal or preoccupation with disturbing emotions or thoughts; mania often causes increased libido.

D. Fear of intimacy may lead to avoidance of all close relationships, while the "madonna/harlot" complex leads to repression of sexual interest in a spouse and sexual activity with another partner. Insight-oriented psychotherapy may help to resolve these conflicts if the patient is willing to stop engaging in extramarital affairs and examine his motivations instead.

E. Change in sexual activity or in interest in a stable partner often signals a more pervasive problem in the relationship.

F. Encourage the couple to discuss their problems openly, explain normal sexual physiology and habits and when appropriate, the effect of the aging process on sexual functioning.

G. A ban is placed on all genital and breast contact, and on intercourse, to help the couple learn to feel comfortable physically with each other. Twenty- to 45–minute "pleasuring sessions" are prescribed at least 3 times per week during which first nonsexual (e.g., touching, massage) and then sexual, contact is structured by the therapist. The couple should tell each other what is pleasurable, and what is not both verbally and by demonstrating how they would like to be touched.

H. Conflict between the feeling that sex is pleasurable and the idea that it is wrong or dirty results in loss of libido. Very gradual introduction of sexual interactions helps focus on the pleasurable aspects of sex without arousing prohibitions against enjoying it and minimizes performance anxiety (pp 114–115).

I. Anxiety, irritability, frustration, missed appointments and failure to carry out assignments indicate discomfort with the couple's current stage of therapy. Since remaining at this stage reinforces negative experiences, the couple should return to the last successful assignment and progress more gradually. Recurrent regressions indicate the need for more intensive discussion of factors such as fears of intimacy, performance anxiety, or undisclosed anger.

J. The couple should spontaneously express an interest in progressing to intercourse before the therapist recommends that they proceed to this step. If they do not but are otherwise functioning better sexually, they should be asked if they feel uncomfortable about the prospect of intercourse.

K. As the couple acquires increasing independence from the therapist, they should increasingly direct their own sexual activities with a gradually decreasing frequency of sessions to monitor for setbacks.

REFERENCES

Masters W, Johnson V. Human Sexual Inadequacy. Boston: Little, Brown, 1970.

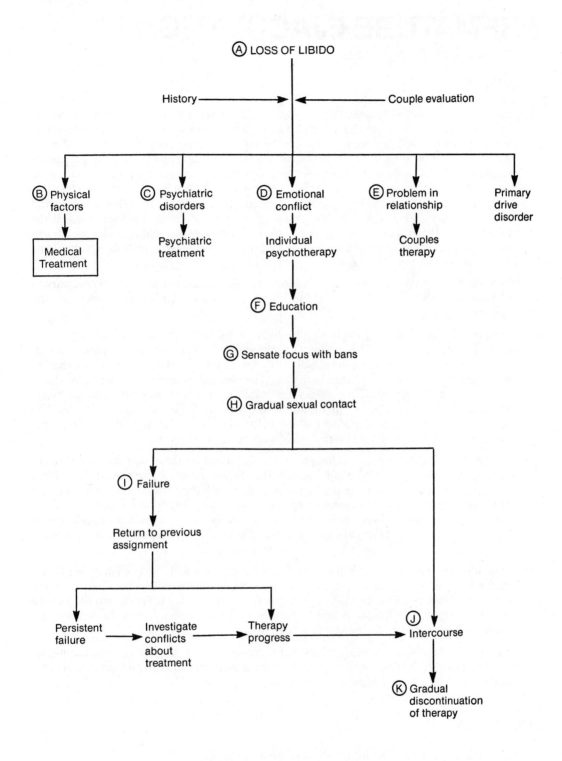

(A) LOSS OF LIBIDO

History ⟶ ⟵ Couple evaluation

(B) Physical factors

Medical Treatment

(C) Psychiatric disorders

Psychiatric treatment

(D) Emotional conflict

Individual psychotherapy

(F) Education

(G) Sensate focus with bans

(H) Gradual sexual contact

(I) Failure

Return to previous assignment

Persistent failure ⟶ Investigate conflicts about treatment ⟶ Therapy progress ⟶ (J) Intercourse

(K) Gradual discontinuation of therapy

(E) Problem in relationship

Couples therapy

Primary drive disorder

Kaplan HS. The New Sex Therapy. New York: Brunner/Mazel, 1974.
Kaplan HS. Disorders of Sexual Desire. New York: Brunner/Mazel, 1974.
Spark J. Impotence is not always psychogenic. JAMA 1980; 243:750–755.

PREMATURE EJACULATION
Daniel A. Hoffman, M.D.

COMMENTS

A. Ejaculation is preceded by a distinctly recognizable sensation (point of ejaculatory inevitability) that heralds the inevitable approach of orgasm. If stimulation is ceased before this point, ejaculation will not occur. Premature ejaculation is currently defined according to whether the couple considers it a problem. Illnesses and medications causing premature ejaculation are discussed on pp 118–119. The couple's expectations of intercourse should be discussed and misconceptions (e.g., that the only "good" orgasm in a woman is produced by intercourse and is prevented by the man's climaxing first) should be dispelled. Amount and type of foreplay and time and circumstances of intercourse should be determined. If the circumstances under which intercourse occurs are conducive to rapid climax (e.g., anxiety about being heard by others in the house or little time for sexual play), an attempt should be made to restructure the setting.

B. The goal of therapy for premature ejaculation is to raise the level of stimulation necessary to produce orgasm. As with all sexual dysfunctions, a ban is placed on intercourse until the orgasmic response is retrained.

C. Techniques used to raise the orgasmic threshold are initially practiced individually by the male, utilizing the approach he prefers. During the stop/start technique, the patient stimulates himself to just before the point of ejaculatory inevitability and then ceases masturbation until the erection recedes at least halfway. The squeeze technique also employs self-stimulation to the point of ejaculatory inevitability, at which point the patient exerts sufficient pressure on the penis with his thumb and first two fingers to decrease arousal. The erection is allowed to recede at least halfway before the process is repeated. The stop/start and squeeze techniques should be repeated 5 or 6 times per session.

D. The stop/start or the squeeze technique is now practiced by the couple with the woman applying the stimulation. If the couple chooses the squeeze technique, the woman should face the man and place her thumb on the frenulum just beneath the coronal ridge on the ventral surface of the penis and her first two fingers above and below the coronal ridge on the dorsal surface. Strong pressure, using the other hand, too, if necessary is exerted until ejaculation no longer feels imminent. As in individual practice, the technique is repeated 5 or 6 times per session.

E. Intercourse should first occur in the female-superior position with the woman on her knees, inserting the penis, and the man controlling thrusting with his hands on her hips. When the point of ejaculatory inevitability is approached the man removes his penis and the woman applies the squeeze technique if that approach has been chosen. When the erection has receded at least halfway, the process is repeated.

F. Even if formal therapy is terminated, the couple must continue to practice these techniques for 6 to 12 months before sexual physiology is completely retrained and intercourse in other positions can be resumed without recurrence of the problem.

REFERENCES

Masters W, Johnson V. Human Sexual Inadequacy. Boston: Little, Brown, 1970.
Kaplan HS. The New Sex Therapy. New York: Brunner/Mazel, 1974.
Kaplan HS. Disorders of Sexual Desire. New York: Brunner/Mazel, 1974.
Spark J. Impotence is not always psychogenic. JAMA 1980; 243:750–755.

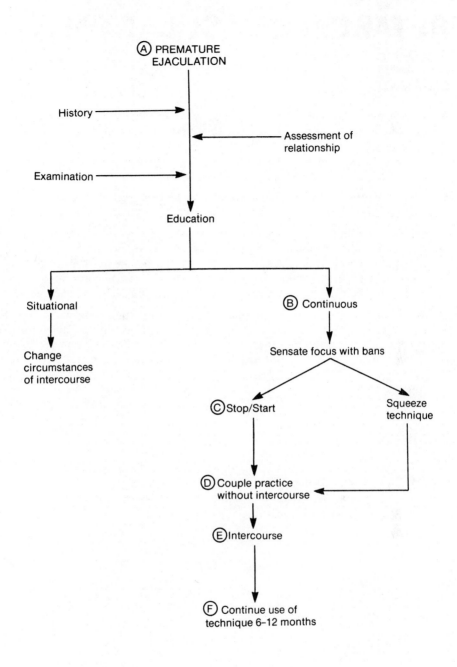

RETARDED EJACULATION

Daniel A. Hoffman, M.D.

COMMENTS

A. Retarded ejaculation, may occur during any sexual activity and is characterized by difficulty proceeding beyond the point of ejaculatory inevitability to intercourse. Illnesses and medications that may cause this problem are discussed on pp 118–119. When it is psychogenic, retarded ejaculation frequently is due to anxiety generated by some aspect of the sexual situation, e.g., fear of the vagina, conflicts, or anger with the partner.

B. Psychotherapy should accompany sex therapy when psychological or marital conflicts are apparent and the patient and his partner are able to discuss them openly.

C. Sex therapy is intended to desensitize the patient to the sexual situation (usually intercourse) that presumably is causing his anxiety. Initially, using any acceptable form of stimulation, the man places his penis outside but near the vagina when he reaches the point of ejaculatory inevitability. After he is able to ejaculate comfortably in greater physical proximity to the vagina, he begins to insert the penis after the point of ejaculatory inevitability.

D. After he becomes accustomed to ejaculating inside the vagina, the man inserts his penis just before reaching the point of ejaculatory inevitability and continues intercourse to ejaculation. If he is able to proceed to orgasm, insertion can occur sooner and previously acceptable sexual activities may be reinstituted. If difficulty in continuing to orgasm returns at any point, the preceding stage should be reinstituted and therapy should proceed more slowly (pp 122–123).

REFERENCES

Masters W, Johnson V. Human Sexual Inadequacy. Boston: Little, Brown, 1970.

Kaplan HS. The New Sex Therapy. New York: Brunner/Mazel, 1974.

Kaplan HS. Disorders of Sexual Desire. New York: Brunner/Mazel, 1974.

Spark J. Impotence is not always psychogenic. JAMA 1980; 243:750–755.

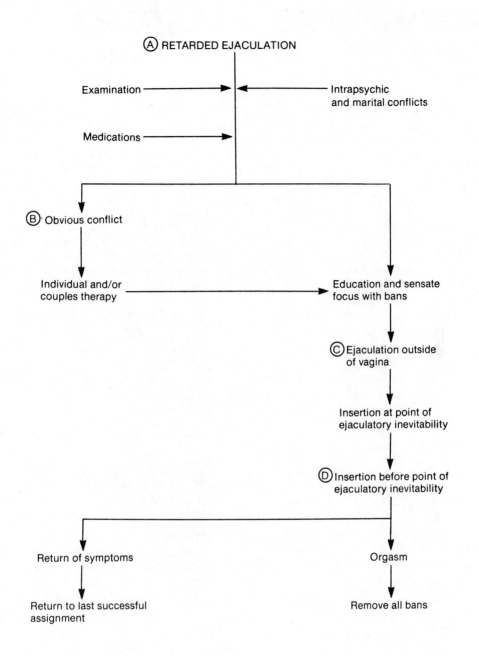

DEVIANT SEXUAL BEHAVIOR

Deborah A. Coyle, M.D.

COMMENTS

A. Sexual deviations (paraphilias) are characterized by the need for unusual, bizarre or deviant stimuli for sexual excitement and inability to achieve sexual satisfaction without the paraphilic object. Many patients are brought to the physician's attention by the family or authorities, since they tend not to regard themselves as ill. Most reported cases involve males. Types of paraphilias include: *fetishism*: use of inanimate objects not designed for sexual purposes as a preferred or exclusive means of achieving sexual stimulation; *transvestism*: persistent dressing in women's clothes for the purpose of sexual excitement; in contrast to the transsexual (pp 166–167), the transvestite has a masculine sexual identity and is heterosexual; *zoophilia*: sexual preference for an animal; *pedophilia*: the act or fantasy of sexual activity with prepubertal children is the preferred or exclusive means of sexual excitement; *exhibitionism*: the patient repeatedly exposes his genitals to a stranger to achieve sexual excitement but with no further sexual activity; *voyeurism*: observation of others who are undressing, naked, or engaging in sexual activity, in order to become sexually aroused; *sexual masochism*: being bound, beaten, humiliated, or otherwise made to suffer is a preferred means of sexual excitement; *sexual sadism*: the need to inflict psychological or physical suffering to achieve sexual excitement.

B. Deviant sexual behavior may be a symptom of organic brain disease, especially dementias, mental retardation, seizure disorders, and intoxication. Psychiatric disorders that can produce paraphilias include schizophrenia, depression, and personality disorders. Sexual deviancy may appear transiently in response to marital discord; it is likely to produce significant marital problems if it persists.

C. Alcohol and illicit drugs decrease control of destructive sexual impulses. Limitation of their use is an essential component of treatment.

D. If pedophilia results in child abuse or neglect, it must be reported to appropriate authorities in most states. If a specific potential victim is identified, it is necessary to warn that person as well as the police. Consultation with a forensic specialist to determine the limits of confidentiality is advisable if the patient reveals that he has injured or raped someone.

E. If impulse control cannot be improved in the patient, the family needs advice about monitoring his behavior and assistance in understanding the limitations of therapy and in adjusting to a permanent personality change. The motivations of a spouse who remains with a recalcitrant sexually deviant patient should be explored.

F. The patient who feels guilty, ashamed, or otherwise uncomfortable about his behavior may benefit from intensive treatment. Conjoint treatment, sex therapy, expressive psychotherapy, antidepressants, or antianxiety drugs should be used if sexual deviance develops in response to an acute marital or sexual problem, depression, or anxiety. Sexual dysfunctions that are not reactive to a situational or psychiatric disturbance are difficult to treat. Therapy involves obtaining a detailed history of behavior and feelings that precede deviant episodes and teaching ways of recognizing and avoiding high risk situations. Negative reinforcement for fantasies about deviant behavior and group therapy may be useful.

REFERENCES

American Psychiatric Association: Diagnostic and Statistical Manual of Mental Disorders. 3rd ed. Washington, DC: American Psychiatric Press, 1980.

Wahl CW. Sexual Problems: Diagnosis and Treatment in Medical Practice. New York: Free Press, 1967.

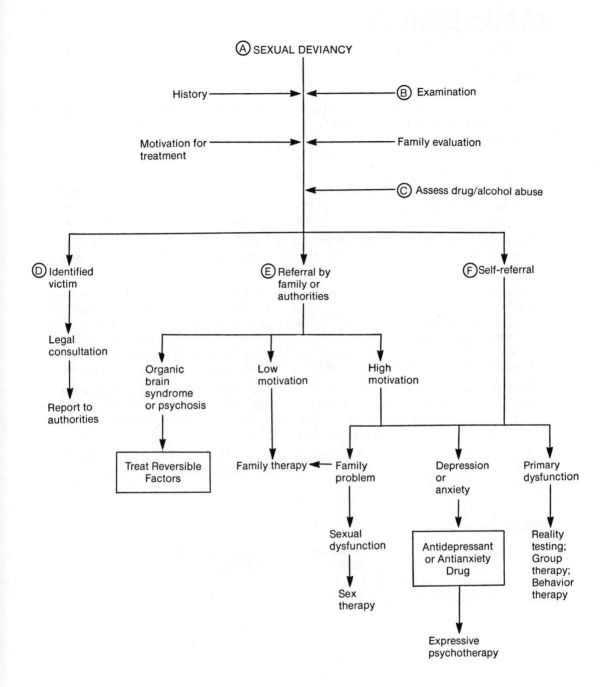

SEXUAL DEVIANCY

A SEXUAL DEVIANCY

History ——→ ←—— B Examination

Motivation for ——→ ←—— Family evaluation
treatment

←—— C Assess drug/alcohol abuse

D Identified victim

E Referral by family or authorities

F Self-referral

Legal consultation

Report to authorities

Organic brain syndrome or psychosis

Low motivation

High motivation

Treat Reversible Factors

Family therapy ←— Family problem

Depression or anxiety

Primary dysfunction

Sexual dysfunction

Antidepressant or Antianxiety Drug

Reality testing; Group therapy; Behavior therapy

Sex therapy

Expressive psychotherapy

VAGINISMUS
Daniel A. Hoffman, M.D.

COMMENTS

A. Vaginismus is a relatively uncommon sexual dysfunction characterized by involuntary muscle spasm preventing penetration. It may be produced by dyspareunia of any cause, previous sexual trauma, or less commonly, by unconscious conflicts about sexuality. If severe, it may physiologically inhibit excitement and orgasm, resulting in failure to lubricate or inability to experience orgasm.

B. As is true of the treatment of most sexual dysfunctions, performance anxiety is reduced by placing a ban on intercourse while helping the woman to focus on the pleasurable aspects of lovemaking and to ignore fears of experiencing vaginismus.

C. The vagina is desensitized by gradually introducing catheters of progressively larger diameter several times per day. The catheter remains in place for at least one-half hour, so that spasms cease before it is removed.

D. Desensitization to aspects of the sexual encounter other than penetration occurs by instructing the partner to insert dilators of gradually increasing size during physical pleasuring sessions. The catheter should remain in place for at least one-half hour while sensate focus (communication of pleasurable and unpleasurable nongenital contact) proceeds. When the woman is able to tolerate dilator insertion without spasm the partner gradually inserts his finger for increasing lengths of time, at first without any attempt to produce excitement.

E. Orgasm is now allowed through manual or oral stimulation. Then, penetration without active thrusting is allowed, in the female-superior position, to produce containment of the penis without any discomfort. When the woman feels comfortable, active intercourse is resumed and all bans eventually are removed.

F. As with the treatment of all sexual dysfunctions, discomfort or failure at any particular stage indicates that therapy is progressing too rapidly and that the couple should return to the preceding successful stage.

REFERENCES

Masters W, Johnson V. Human Sexual Inadequacy. Boston: Little, Brown, 1970.
Kaplan HS. The New Sex Therapy. New York: Brunner/Mazel, 1974.
Kaplan HS. Disorders of Sexual Desire. New York: Brunner/Mazel, 1974.
Spark J. Impotence is not always psychogenic. JAMA 1980; 243:750–755.

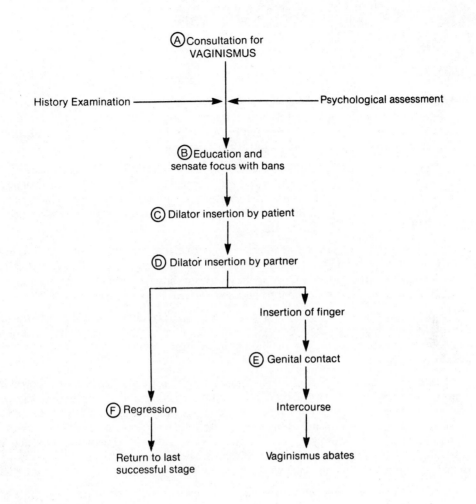

History Examination ⟶ Ⓐ Consultation for VAGINISMUS ⟵ Psychological assessment

Ⓑ Education and sensate focus with bans

Ⓒ Dilator insertion by patient

Ⓓ Dilator insertion by partner

Insertion of finger

Ⓔ Genital contact

Ⓕ Regression

Intercourse

Return to last successful stage

Vaginismus abates

ANOREXIA NERVOSA
Robert M. House, M.D.

COMMENTS

A. Anorexia nervosa is a chronic, potentially fatal (4 to 10%), self-imposed state of starvation of unknown cause with onset in adolescence or young adulthood. It affects women 20 times as frequently as men and is characterized by loss of more than 25 percent of ideal weight, conviction of being obese, and compulsive physical exercise.

B. Malignancies, anemias, vitamin deficiencies, parasitic infections, and other causes of starvation may mimic anorexia nervosa but are not usually associated with a disordered body image. Depression may be associated with lack of interest in food, while obsessive-compulsive patients may develop ritualistic diets and schizophrenics may have delusional fears of food leading to self-starvation.

C. Despite her emaciation, the anorectic patient may feel that her only problem is that she needs to lose a little more weight. If she is competent and not in immediate danger, she cannot be forced to accept therapy (pp 142–143); the physician should attempt to establish a supportive relationship and allow the patient to determine when she would like to begin therapy.

D. Hospitalization may become necessary to correct electrolyte imbalance and dehydration and provide hyperalimentation. If the patient whose life is in danger refuses, therapy, hospitalization should be arranged. Once the patient is stabilized, transfer to an inpatient psychiatric setting is indicated.

E. Attempts to coerce the patient into attaining a normal weight are likely to reproduce the power struggle over eating and control. Psychotherapy cannot be helpful until the biologic effects of starvation have been reversed. Behavior modification may be necessary if the patient cannot maintain her weight at a safe level. The patient should be involved in formulating the behavior program which usually includes reward with unlimited activity for weight gain and restriction of activity and other reinforcers if the patient does not gain a specified amount of weight each week.

F. Outpatient therapy can be considered when the patient is able to maintain a stable weight. Psychological issues include denial of the need for treatment, a sense of ineffectiveness dealt with by maintaining exact control over body weight in defiance of others' wishes, and difficulty in establishing independence and self-esteem. Struggles over the patient's weight should be avoided unless it falls below an agreed upon level, in which case she should be rehospitalized.

G. Most anorectic patients suffer from conflicts with their families over control, independence, and separation. Family therapy can help them resolve these conflicts.

H. Depression may be an additional problem in patients who become suicidal or have a past history or family history of affective disorder or response to antidepressants. Other signs of depression such as guilt, insomnia, appetite change, decreased interest in sex, and change in activity do not distinguish reliably between anorexia and depression. Antidepressants should be used with great caution in patients with cardiovascular instability due to starvation.

REFERENCES

Barcai A. Family therapy in the treatment of anorexia nervosa. Amer J Psychiatry 1971; 128:286–290.

Bruch H. Anorexia nervosa: therapy and theory. Amer J Psychiatry 1982; 139:1531–1538.

Bruch H. Eating Disorders: Obesity, Anorexia Nervosa, and the Person Within. New York: Basic Books, 1973.

Eckert ED, Goldberg SC, Halmi KA, et al. Behavior therapy in anorexia nervosa. Br J Psychiatry 1979; 134:55–59.

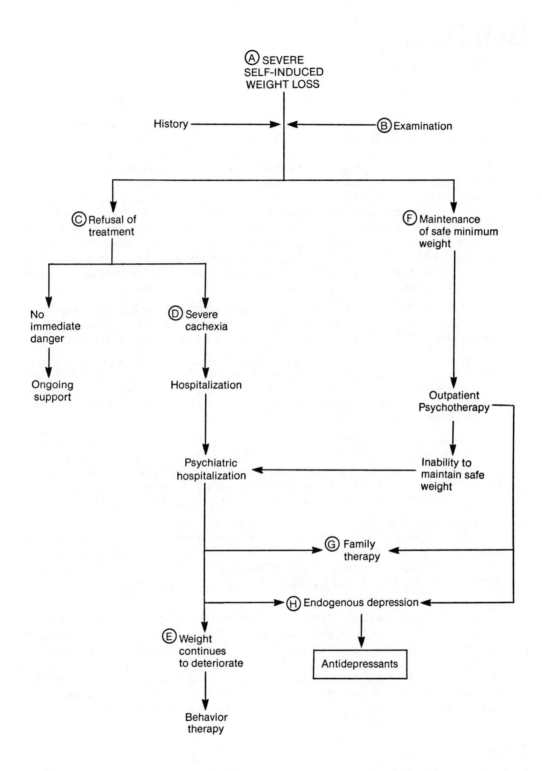

Moore DC. Amitriptyline therapy in anorexia nervosa. Amer J Psychiatry 1977; 134:1303–1304.

BULIMIA

Robert M. House, M.D.

COMMENTS

A. Patients with bulimia episodically eat large quantities of high-calorie food one or more times per day, often in secret. Because of abdominal discomfort, guilt, or fear that they will not be able to stop eating, they terminate eating binges with self-induced vomiting and/or laxative abuse. This disorder is seen primarily in adolescent girls and young women, especially in college populations. Some patients with antisocial lifestyles are prone to bulimia. Like the patient with anorexia nervosa, the bulimic is preoccupied with food and body weight; however, appetite is normal, weight tends to fluctuate on either side of a fairly stable baseline, and the patient has a realistic body image. Bulimics are more extroverted and have a greater interest in sex than anorectics. Medical conditions that may be associated with symptoms similar to bulimia include hyperthyroidism, central nervous system tumors (especially of the hypothalamus), Klein-Levin syndrome, Kluver-Bucy syndrome, schizophrenia, and use of oral contraceptives.

B. Physical complications that may result include electrolyte imbalance and dehydration from vomiting and laxative abuse, dental caries caused by acidic content of vomitus, Mallory-Weiss syndrome and bilateral, painless, benign parotid enlargement of unknown cause.

C. The patient who is discovered during a purging episode and is brought to a physician by others may visit the doctor to please them but have little interest in changing her behavior. The bulimic patient is often afraid of losing control; she should not be coerced into treatment. Ongoing availability to the patient may allow her to seek therapy when it feels like her decision rather than someone else's.

D. In recent years, young women have felt intense social pressure to remain thin; but some who cannot suppress their appetites vomit in an attempt to keep from gaining weight. Their bulimic behavior often remits spontaneously when the social situation changes. Education about the ineffectiveness of this method of weight control and its potential adverse effects, and counseling about more effective methods may help the patient alter her behavior.

E. The bulimic patient finds it difficult to deal with anxiety, sadness, helplessness, anger, and conflicts over dependency. Purging after eating temporarily helps relieve the fear that her eating is out of control, but guilt, disgust, and loss of control ensue. The goal of individual or group psychotherapy is to provide the patient with a greater sense of mastery by allowing her to deal with conflicts more directly. Bulimia tends to be recurrent or chronic; treatment is often prolonged.

F. Symptoms of depression such as sleep disturbance, diurnal mood swing, guilt, and lowered self-esteem indicate a trial of antidepressant medication. Antidepressants, particularly imipramine and trazodone, may also be an effective adjunctive treatment for patients without obvious depression, especially if psychotherapy alone is ineffective. Patients who do not respond to psychotherapy and antidepressants may experience a decrease in binging when they take tranylcypromine or phenelzine. It is crucial to be certain that the indiscriminate eater avoids foods containing tyramine before prescribing an MAO inhibitor.

REFERENCES

Casper RC, Eckert ED, Halmi KA, Goldberg SC, Davis JM. Bulimia. Arch Gen Psychiatry 1980; 37:1030–1035.

Gwirtsman HE, Roy-Byrne P, Yoger J, Gerner RH. Neuroendocrine abnormalities in bulimia. Amer J Psychiatry 1983; 140:558–563.

Herzog DB. Bulimia: The secrective syndrome. Psychosomatics 1982; 23:481–487.

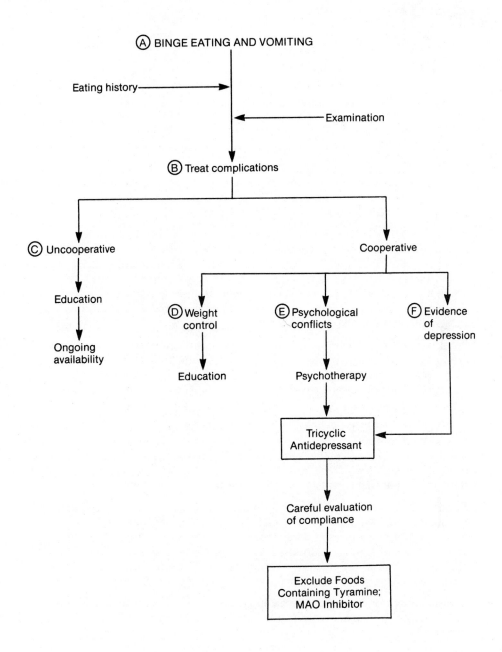

Ⓐ BINGE EATING AND VOMITING

Eating history

Examination

Ⓑ Treat complications

Ⓒ Uncooperative

Education

Ongoing availability

Cooperative

Ⓓ Weight control

Education

Ⓔ Psychological conflicts

Psychotherapy

Ⓕ Evidence of depression

Tricyclic Antidepressant

Careful evaluation of compliance

Exclude Foods Containing Tyramine; MAO Inhibitor

Johnson C, Berndt DJ. Preliminary investigation of bulimia and life adjustment. Amer J Psychiatry 1983; 140:774–777.

Pope HG, Hudson JI, Jonas JM, Yurgelun-Tod D. Bulimia treated with imipramine: a placebo-controlled, double blind study. Amer J Psychiatry 1983; 140:554–558.

OBESITY

Robert M. House, M.D. and Wendy L. Thompson, M.D.

COMMENTS

A. Eighty million Americans are at least 10 percent overweight, and one-fourth of Americans are more than 10 kilograms over their ideal weight. Morbid obesity (weight greater than 100% of ideal body weight) is less common. Loss of weight may not mean loss of fat; accurate measures of body fat should be made and followed during therapy.

B. Investigate age of onset of weight gain, family history of obesity, eating habits, psychological significance of food and weight, and previous attempts at weight loss. Complications such as diabetes mellitus, hypertension, alveolar hypoventilation syndrome (Pickwickian syndrome), sleep apnea, and multiple orthopedic problems are unlikely to be problematic until the patient is more than 20 to 30 percent overweight.

C. Edema and pregnancy can produce weight gain. Organic causes of obesity, which are present in 5 percent of cases, include rare congenital disorders such as Laurence-Moon-Biedl Syndrome, hyperostosis frontalis interna, and Prader-Willi Syndrome, CNS and endocrine problems (Cushing's syndrome). Older, previously active patients who become sedentary may also become obese. Medications that may stimulate weight gain include adrenal steroids, tricyclic antidepressants, and oral contraceptives.

D. Professional athletes who intentionally gain weight are not necessarily "obese"; a large proportion of their bulk is muscle. They need to be taught that continued high caloric intake with decreased activity will lead to obesity. Members of some cultures value obesity; empathy, education and nutritional counseling may be helpful to them.

E. Most people do not gain weight purposely and weight loss may be very difficult. Depression may cause weight gain by affecting hypothalamic function or by decreasing activity. Food may be used to relieve negative feelings or to avoid intimacy. If the patient's psychological resources are so limited that anxiety resulting from weight loss would be too disturbing and overall functioning would be more likely to be preserved by remaining overweight, gradual strengthening of the patient's defences must precede weight loss.

F. Characteristics of a successful weight loss program include: (1) diet suited to the patient's preference and lifestyle with realistic goals, (2) high patient interest, (3) aerobic exercise to maintain lean body mass and enhance metabolism of calories, (4) encouragement from family and peers, (5) diary of food intake and exercise to identify problem areas of which the patient is unaware, (6) change of eating habits. Appetite suppressants may be useful in producing short-term loss that encourages the patient but lose their effectiveness rapidly.

G. Longstanding obesity may serve an important psychological function within the family; significant weight loss may require psychotherapy to help establish a new equilibrium for the family.

H. Surgical approaches produce lasting weight loss (about 60% of excess body weight) that often improves the depression and psychosocial problems associated with morbid obesity; however, the risk is not justified in patients with only moderate obesity. Jejunoileal bypass carries a much greater risk of medical complications (especially electrolyte imbalance, liver and renal disease) than do gastric bypass and gastroplasty. In addition to decreased food intake to avoid diarrhea or vomiting, operations for surgery seem to reset the appetite mechanism.

I. Group counseling may be helpful to patients who have undergone surgery for obesity. Ongoing peer support and encouragement to continue the weight loss effort are also helpful.

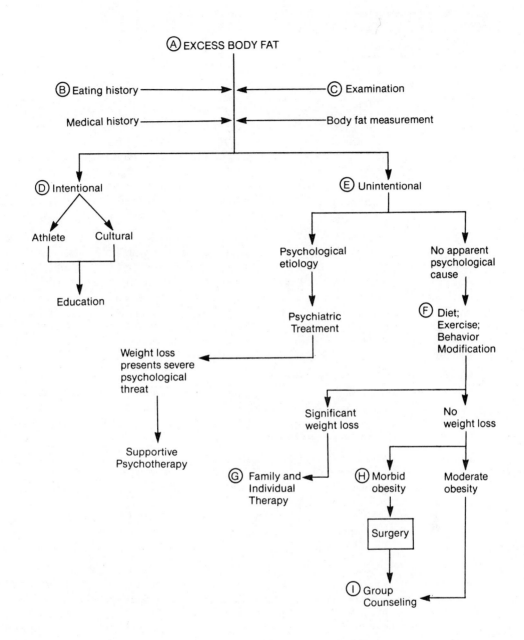

REFERENCES

Bruch H. Eating Disorders: Obesity, Anorexia Nervosa and the Person Within. New York: Basic Books, 1973.

Levitz LS, Stunkard AJ. A therapeutic coalition for obesity: behavior modification and patient self-help. Amer J Psychiat 1974; 131:423–427.

Powers P. Obesity. Psychosomatics 1982; 23:1023–1039.

Rand CSW, Stunkard AJ. Obesity and Psychoanalysis. Amer J Psychiat 1978; 135:547–551.

Stunkard AJ, Penik SB. Behavior modification in the treatment of obesity; the problem of maintaining weight loss. Arch Gen Psychiat 1979; 36:801–806.

Wolman BB. Psychologic Aspects of Obesity: A Handbook. New York: Van Nostrand Reinhold, 1982.

ANTISOCIAL PERSONALITY

Neil Baker, M.D.

COMMENTS

A. Antisocial *behavior* may accompany mania, schizophrenia, personality disorders, substance abuse, organic brain syndromes, and mental retardation. Antisocial *personality disorder* is a specific syndrome characterized by onset of multiple antisocial behaviors before age 15. Unlawful behavior continues into adult life, as do inability to maintain a job, relationship problems, failure to pay debts, poor impulse control, low frustration tolerance, impulsivity, substance abuse, disregard for social norms, inability to learn from experience, and a tendency to relieve anxiety through action. Relationships tend to be shallow, coercive, and demanding. Any stressor that interferes with outlets for action may produce psychological or behavioral symptoms.

B. The general psychiatric history should be supplemented by an investigation of: current stresses that might lead to malingering; impulsivity; legal and work history; and violent and suicidal thoughts and behavior. The patient with antisocial personality tends to disregard the truth; questioning must be specific and the physician assertive in pursuing the history, contacting other informants for corroboration. If the physician meets his needs, the patient may appear sincere and cooperative, resulting in the physician's minimizing the patient's psychopathology. Coercive, demanding, and dishonest behavior when the patient is not gratified may make the physician feel angry, helpless, disgusted, or demoralized.

C. Patients with antisocial personality may shout, threaten or destroy property in order to simulate illness, express disappointment, coerce favors, or indirectly request controls. Unacceptable behaviors should be clearly identified, and their consequences stated and adhered to strictly. Persistent agitation requires restraint and/or sedation. If the patient is potentially dangerous, guidelines on pp 24–25 apply.

D. Disruptive behavior or coercive demands increase if the physician does not confront the underlying motivation which may be quick relief of anxiety or manipulation of the physician. The physician must avoid acceding to inappropriate demands so that the patient does not learn to control him through destructive interactions. Attempts should be made to identify and find better solutions to the problems that led to the patient's symptoms. If disruptive behavior or demands persist, further treatment should be offered only when he is able to control his behavior.

E. Depression and anxiety occur when the patient's usual means of manipulating his environment are ineffective and his behavior restricted. He should be told that, while drugs will not be prescribed and/or jail avoided, some distress may be alleviated by talking. The physician should help identify the precipitating stress and maladaptive responses, survey previous means of handling difficulties, and find better ways of dealing with unpleasant emotions. Signs of endogenous depression warrant a trial antidepressant. If the patient improves and wishes more treatment, long-term psychotherapy should focus on present reality and problem solving rather than affects, fantasies, and the past.

F. Previously controlled antisocial traits that are a patient's principle means of reducing anxiety may be exacerbated by intercurrent psychoses, depression, or organic brain syndromes.

REFERENCES

Reid WH. The Treatment of Antisocial Syndromes. New York: Van Nostrand Reinhold Co, 1981.
Lion JR. Personality Disorders: Diagnosis and Management. Baltimore: Williams & Wilkins, 1981.
Cleckley H. The Mask of Sanity. 5th ed. St. Louis: CV Mosby, 1975.

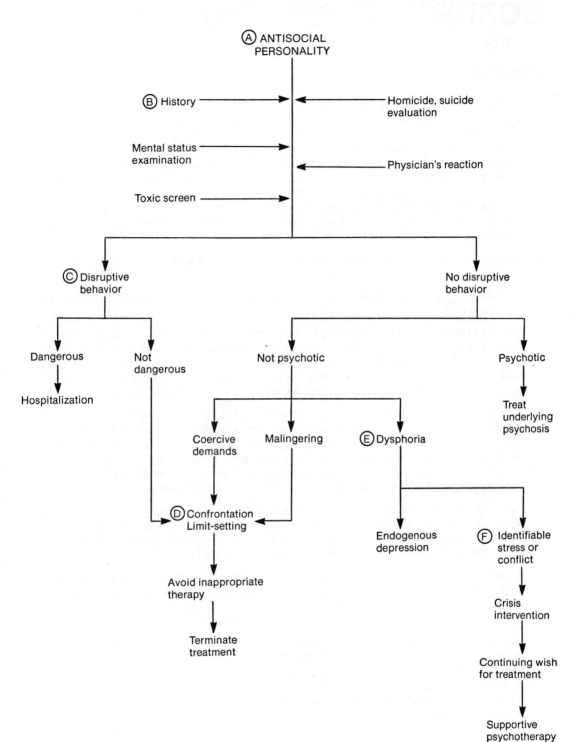

BORDERLINE PERSONALITY

Troy L. Thompson II, M.D. and Michael G. Moran, M.D.

COMMENTS

A. Patients with superficially good adaptation who become disorganized in response to certain kinds of stress, especially in intense interpersonal relationships, may have a borderline personality organization. Although some have considered it a form of schizophrenia, this syndrome is now regarded as a personality disorder that lies between neurosis and psychosis. The diagnosis is suggested by disordered relationships, multiple neurotic symptoms, chronic feelings of emptiness, intolerance of being alone, drug abuse, promiscuity, suicide attempts, identity disturbance, and transient psychotic symptoms. Patients with borderline personality experience psychological disorganization, low self-esteem, fears of rejection, intense anger, self-destructive behavior, and at times, psychosis, whenever any relationship becomes too intimate or too distant.

B. Physicians frequently feel puzzled, frustrated, and angry in response to the provocative and changeable behavior of such patients.

C. Features suggesting major depression improve the prognosis for overall adaptation and warrant a trial of antidepressant therapy.

D. Hostility may represent an attempt to distance himself from a person with whom the patient feels he is becoming too intimate, an attempt at manipulation, or a derivative of feelings originally directed toward inadequate caregivers. Less frequent but regular appointments and less intensive discussions may help decrease his hostility. Confronting rage that the patient projects and denies is an essential component of expressive psychotherapy.

E. The patient is likely to become more frightened and angry and to further test him if the physician fails to prohibit all destructive behavior. The physician should discontinue the relationship with a patient who persists in frightening or disruptive behavior directed to him. Necessary medical care can be provided by emergency or clinic services. If the patient is able to talk about negative feelings without acting on them and is interested in examining longstanding conflicts, he may benefit from more intensive psychotherapy.

F. Splitting refers to contradictory but concurrent emotional states and ideas. One result is that some people develop unrealistically positive attitudes toward the patient while others feel the opposite because the patient feels and behaves differently with different people. This may be minimized if all involved discuss the treatment plan regularly.

G. Demands for medications often reflect a wish to be soothed, to receive something concrete, or to manipulate and test the physician. Demands for potentially addicting substances are likely to escalate once a drug is prescribed. Low doses of nonsedating antipsychotic drugs such as haloperidol or thiothixene may lessen intolerable anxiety.

H. Self-limited paranoia, suicidal and homicidal feelings, and hallucinations may develop in reaction to a change in the physician's attitude. If dysphoria or disturbed behavior do not remit with limit-setting, discussion of feelings that provoked decompensation, and increased structure in the doctor-patient relationship, brief (1–14 days) hospitalization is indicated. To obviate further decompensation, the patient should be told in advance that his hospitalization will be brief.

REFERENCES

Beresin E, Gordon C. Emergency ward management of the borderline patient. Gen Hosp Psychiatry 1981; 3:237–244.

Dubovsky SL. Psychotherapeutics in Primary Care. New York: Grune & Stratton, 1981: 115–151.

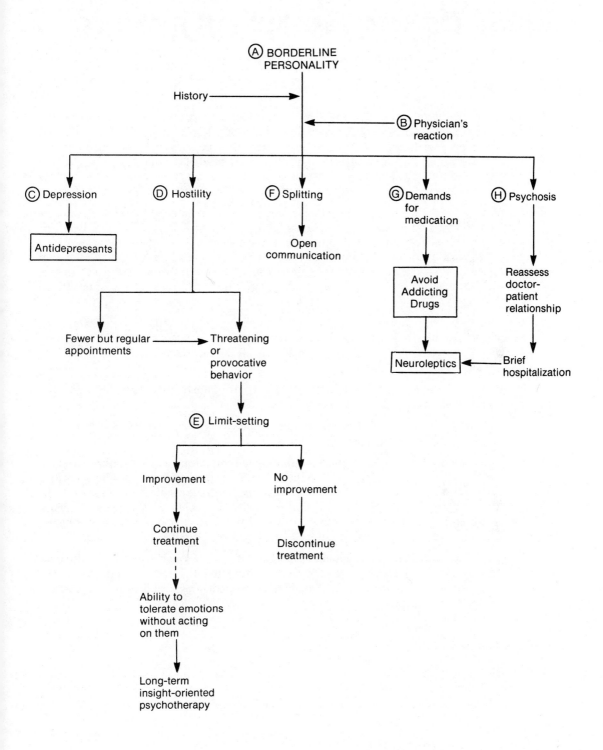

Groves JE. Management of the borderline patient on a medical or surgical ward: the psychiatric consultant's role. Internat J Psychiatry Med 1975; 6:337–348.

Groves JE. Borderline personality disorder. New Engl J Med 1981; 305(5):259–262.

Gunderson JG, Singer MT. Defining borderline patients: an overview. Amer J Psychiatry 1975; 132:1.

CIVIL COMMITMENT OF ADULTS

Jeffrey L. Metzner, M.D.

COMMENTS

A. Many seriously ill patients who initially refuse hospitalization see the need for inpatient care after they are admitted. Criteria for involuntary hospitalization of patients vary greatly, and the following guidelines are general. Commitment may be sought for patients who are suffering from a mental illness that causes them to be: in need of treatment; gravely disabled and unable to care for their basic needs; or dangerous to themselves or others. Most states require "clear and convincing" evidence of these criteria (about a 75% level of certainty).

B. The history should be obtained from the patient and other, reliable, sources. The examination should focus on presenting complaints, past psychiatric history, history of behavior dangerous to self or others, mental status examination, information facilitating a psychiatric diagnosis, reasons for refusing hospitalization, current and best level of functioning, and available supports. The diagnosis and treatment plan should be confirmed with a colleague, and the hospital attorney should be asked to verify the correctness of the approach to commitment.

C. If no mental disorder is present, the patient cannot be forced to undergo hospitalization. If a psychiatric disorder associated with dangerousness is unlikely or if there is no clearly specified severe disability, pressures from the family or the physician's reaction may be influencing the treatment plan.

D. Patients who are not certifiable should be offered appropriate treatment and follow-up but permitted to refuse these. Careful records of patient-doctor interactions should be kept.

E. Even though dangerousness cannot always be predicted accurately, high risk (pp 20–21) is sufficient to justify hospitalization.

F. The exact procedures for initiating and continuing civil commitment vary from state to state. In many instances, any physician or the police may initiate proceedings. Consultation with a local attorney is advisable if the physician is unfamiliar with the procedure in his state. If the patient is likely to follow through with appropriate therapy, voluntary treatment is preferable. However, even if the patient agrees to treatment initially, certification should be sought if his behavior is sufficiently erratic to suggest that he may soon refuse to cooperate.

G. The rights of civilly committed patients must be protected through access to an attorney, visits from and communication with others, and the right to refuse treatment. In most states, medications may not be administered to a committed patient against his will unless immediately necessary to protect the patient or someone else.

REFERENCES

Addington v. Texas, 441 U.S. 418 (1979).
Gutheil TG, Appelbaum PS. Clinical Handbook of Psychiatry and Law. New York: McGraw-Hill, 1982.
Grinspoon L. Psychiatry 1982. Washington, DC: American Psychiatric Press, 1982: 334–349.

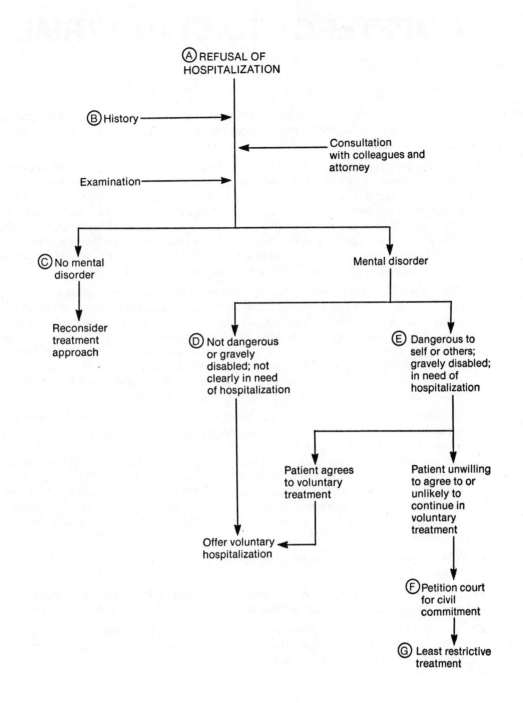

A REFUSAL OF HOSPITALIZATION

B History

Consultation with colleagues and attorney

Examination

C No mental disorder

Mental disorder

Reconsider treatment approach

D Not dangerous or gravely disabled; not clearly in need of hospitalization

E Dangerous to self or others; gravely disabled; in need of hospitalization

Patient agrees to voluntary treatment

Patient unwilling to agree to or unlikely to continue in voluntary treatment

Offer voluntary hospitalization

F Petition court for civil commitment

G Least restrictive treatment

COMPETENCY TO STAND TRIAL

Jeffrey L. Metzner, M.D.

COMMENTS

A. A defendant is legally incompetent to stand trial if he has a mental disorder that significantly impairs his understanding of the legal proceedings or his ability to participate rationally in his own defense. Specific federal and state standards vary.

B. Competency examinations are often requested for a variety of covert reasons. For example, defense attorneys may request an evaluation to assess the possibility of a future insanity plea as a delaying tactic to weaken the prosecution's case or forestall incarceration, or as a step in plea bargaining. Prosecutors may request an evaluation to delay the defendant's release on bail. These evaluations should be expedited by the examiner to minimize future inappropriate referrals. Review of police reports and information about the defendant from other sources will help the examiner prepare for the evaluation. The patient's attorney should be contacted for additional data to determine any covert reasons for referral.

C. The defendant should be fully informed about the purpose of the evaluation and the limits of confidentiality. Complete notes, including relevant verbatim statements of the defendant are essential to the examiner's credibility in court. Before the interview proceeds, the patient's dangerousness should be evaluated (pp 20–21); sufficient staff should be available to ensure the physician's safety. The examination should consist of medical, psychiatric, family, and other pertinent history, details of present illness, discussion of the patient's understanding of the legal proceedings, and mental status examination. A comprehensive battery of psychological tests (pp 176–177) often helps to clarify uncertain findings.

D. If no mental disorder (usually psychosis or organic brain syndrome) is present, the defendant is legally competent. Simulation of mental illness is suggested by: vague, excessively detailed, or spontaneously volunteered descriptions of psychiatric symptoms, especially depression, anxiety, and suicidal thoughts; an expressed desire to be found incompetent; request for mental health treatment; attentiveness to minute details of the examination; inconsistent history; total amnesia for the alleged crime or recall only of specifics that place the defendant in a favorable light; appropriate interactions with people other than the examiner or authorities but inappropriate behavior when under scrutiny; and intimidation of the examiner.

E. Written reports should be free of jargon and should specify the diagnosis, treatment recommendations, and prognosis.

F. It is possible for the patient to be psychotic and still meet the criteria for legal competency if he understands the legal proceedings and is able to participate rationally in his own defense.

G. The report should include the prognosis for restoration of competency. If incompetency is likely to continue indefinitely, the court must institute civil commitment proceedings (pp 142–143) or release the defendant.

REFERENCES

Group for the Advancement of Psychiatry (G.A.P.). Misuse of Psychiatry in the Criminal Courts: Competency to Stand Trial. New York: Group for the Advancement of Psychiatry, 1974.

Lipsitt LD, Lelos D, McGarry AL. Competency for trial: a screening instrument. Amer J Psychiatry 1971; 128:105–109.

Macdonald JM. Psychiatry and the Criminal. Springfield, Illinois: CC Thomas, 1976.

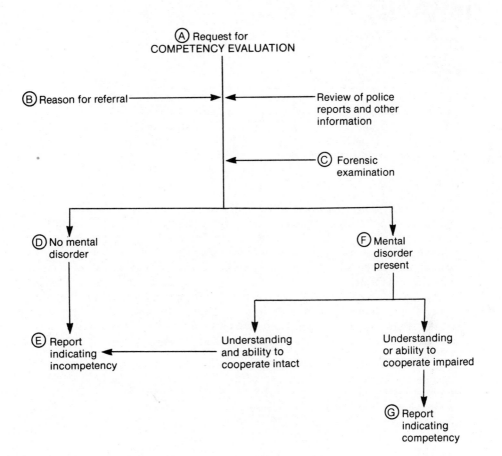

INSANITY PLEA

Jeffrey L. Metzner, M.D.

COMMENTS

A. Since Western law stipulates that a person who is not morally blameworthy for his behavior should not be punished, moral concepts are involved in legal definitions of insanity. Specific legal tests of insanity vary. Physicians who feel that clinically relevant findings cannot be translated accurately into legal tests of insanity should not participate as examiners in insanity evaluations. Psychiatrists who are comfortable in offering opinions regarding the legal issue of sanity must accept that, like experts in any field, they are likely to disagree with each other.

B. Contact with family, friends, witnesses, and victim(s) in addition to a review of all relevant legal documents and past psychiatric reports should be considered in assessing the defendant's state of mind at the time of the alleged crime(s). An insanity evaluation generally requires several interviews; the defendant should be fully informed about the purpose of the evaluation and the limits of confidentiality. Detailed records, including relevant verbatim statements of the defendant, are essential. The evaluation is similar to the standard psychiatric examination but emphasizes in great detail the events pertinent to the alleged crime(s), any personal gain resulting therefrom, and the legal, drug, alcohol, and psychiatric history. Mental status examination should assess paranoid thinking, signs of psychosis, especially command hallucinations, reality testing, and impulse control at the time of the alleged crime.

C. In general, defendants who are too psychotic to participate meaningfully in the evaluation meet the legal criteria for incompetence (pp 144–145) and cannot be tried or evaluated further until competence is restored. The report should state whether the patient is competent or incompetent. If the defendant refuses to cooperate with the examination for reasons unrelated to a mental disorder, the evaluator should state that he cannot offer an opinion based on this examination alone.

D. All commonly used tests for insanity seek to establish whether or not a mental disease or defect at the time of the crime(s) impaired the defendant's ability to behave differently. Although most people who are found not guilty by reason of insanity suffered at the time of the crime from an active severe psychotic mental disorder, most psychotic people do not meet the criteria for legal insanity. The successful use of this defense is rare.

E. If the examination reveals no evidence of a mental disorder at the time of the alleged crime(s), the defendant does not meet the criteria for legal insanity.

F. Defendants whose behavior resulted from the voluntary ingestion of alcohol are legally excluded from using the insanity defense. Exceptions include a first episode of pathological alcohol intoxication and delirium tremens. The American Psychiatric Association statement on the Insanity Defense (1982) recommends that exclusion from the insanity defense be extended to voluntary ingestion of other psychoactive substances.

G. All reports should be organized, free of jargon, and should include a description of the defendant's state of mind at the time of the alleged crime(s), the psychiatric diagnosis, and the examiner's opinion. Clinical findings relied upon and their application to the sanity test should be made clear.

REFERENCES

Gutheil TG, Appelbaum PS. Clinical Handbook of Psychiatry and Law. New York: McGraw-Hill, 1982.
Halleck SL. Law and the Practice of Psychiatry, a Handbook for Clinicians. New York: Plenum Press, 1980.
MacDonald JM. Psychiatry and the Criminal. Springfield, Illinois: CC Thomas, 1976.

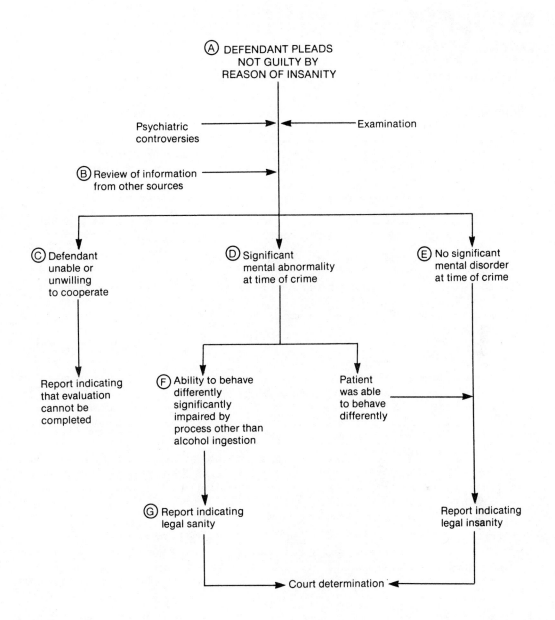

ADOLESCENT SUICIDAL BEHAVIOR

William V. Good, M.D.

COMMENTS

A. The incidence of suicide in adolescents, largely by firearmes, has increased dramatically in recent years. Accident proneness, school failure, fighting, and other forms of self-destructive behavior may be ways of conveying covert suicidal thinking. Suicide in adolescents characteristically is an impulsive reaction to receipt of bad news. Precipitating factors may include: pregnancy, break-up of a relationship, drug abuse, and difficulty in school.

B. Severe psychiatric disorders such as depression, schizophrenia, and organic brain syndrome may produce suicidal behavior in adolescents.

C. While many risk factors for adolescent suicide are the same as for adults additional risk factors may be present in adolescence, including: feeling that death is pleasant or reversible; no other solution to a life situation is apparent; a previous major suicidal attempt has been made; suicidal threats are not an obvious attempt to manipulate the family or environment; propensity to miscalculate risks; serious underlying psychopathology.

D. The goals of hospitalization are protection of the patient, withdrawal of drugs and alcohol, and involvement of the family.

E. Unresolved conflicts that may result in suicidal behavior in reaction to the many normal stresses of adolescence include: difficulty establishing independence; difficulty in establishing cohesive identity, indicated for example, by rapidly shifting peer groups; uncertainty about sexual preference; inability to develop stable peer relations, with absence of friends or association with violence-prone groups.

F. The patient should be examined alone first, and then with the family. If immediate suicidal risk is low, the patient's confidentiality should be protected, but if the adolescent is acutely suicidal or severely disturbed, the family must be informed of the seriousness of the situation. An unsupportive family increases suicidal risk; hospitalization is warranted to protect the patient and to determine why the family is unsupportive.

G. Every effort should be made to involve the family for subsequent supportive assistance. If the family is so angry with the patient that their involvement is likely to be destructive, or if the patient does not want them to be involved, family therapy may need to be deferred. If the family refuses to be evaluated, psychotherapy of the adolescent should be instituted and continued attempts made to involve the family.

H. Continued antagonism or lack of support from the family suggests that the family will be unable to tolerate talking about conflicts without encouraging suicidal behavior in the adolescent. The patient may continue to attempt to free himself from the family by making suicide attempts that result in hospitalization away from the family until his need to be separated from them is recognized.

I. Since suicidal behavior in adolescents often reflects difficulty within the family or attempts to emancipate from them, their involvement is essential to successful therapy. Suicidal ideas are very likely to resolve with the precipitating crisis.

REFERENCES

Holinger PS. Adolescent suicide: an epidemiological study of recent trends. Amer J Psychiatry 1978; 135:525–530.
Miles CP. Conditions predisposing to suicide: a review. J New Ment Dis 1977; 164:231–246.

ADOLESCENT SUICIDAL BEHAVIOR

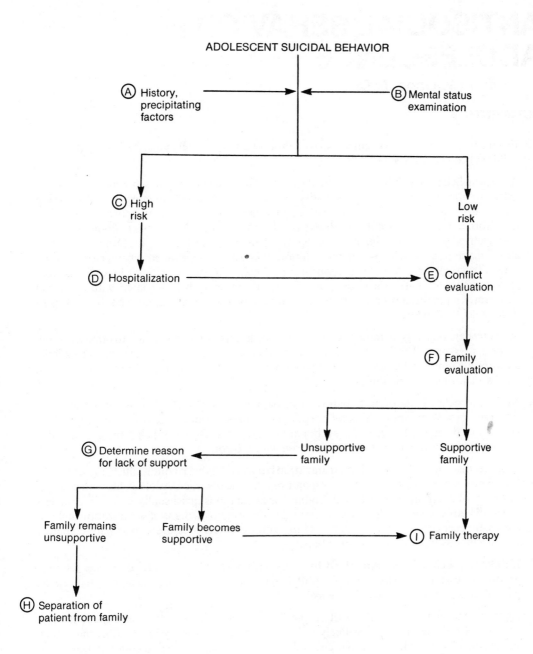

Farley G, Eckhardt L, Hebert FB. Handbook of Child and Adolescent Psychiatric Emergencies. New York: Medical Examination and Publishing, 1979.

ANTISOCIAL BEHAVIOR IN ADOLESCENCE

William V. Good, M.D.

COMMENTS

A. From 5 to 15% of teenagers engage in some sort of antisocial behavior; 35% of all antisocial children become antisocial adults.

B. Antisocial behavior in adolescents may be associated with depression, schizophrenia, hyperactivity, substance abuse, and personality disorders. Adolescents are more likely to develop antisocial behavior when there is disruption or violence in the family, an antisocial personality disorder in either parent, an absent or alcoholic father, low socioeconomic status, a disorganized social environment, or parental acceptance of such behavior. Drug and alcohol abuse make antisocial behavior more likely. It must be determined whether drug abuse causes behavior or is a manifestation of a personality disorder. Frontal lobe disease and seizure disorders, particularly temporal lobe epilepsy, may be associated with antisocial behavior. Generalized organic brain syndromes may also impair impulse control and produce violent behavior.

C. Many teenagers engage in minor victimless antisocial acts, often in reaction to family, school, or peer pressures. The behavior is likely to resolve spontaneously if the patient exhibits appropriate remorse, comes from an intact, nonviolent and nonabusing family, and does not have a major psychiatric illness.

D. Antisocial behavior is often a symptom of depression, especially if it is self-destructive. Adolescents with paranoid thinking are prone to aggressive antisocial behavior; schizophrenia may be disguised by "pseudopsychopathic" behavior. Depressed children who are also antisocial have a worse prognosis than those who are not.

E. Conduct disorder is diagnosed when antisocial behavior has been continuously present for at least 6 months in the absence of other major psychiatric disorder. Adolescents with conduct disorder who are able to establish stable social relationships usually come from a less disruptive environment and have a better long-term prognosis. Signs of socialization include: consistent peer group; antisocial behavior in response to peer pressure; capacity for empathy; warm relationships with family members.

F. If antisocial behavior is encouraged by peers, efforts should be made to change the peer group. Group therapy may be very helpful. Ongoing encouragement is necessary to keep the patient away from destructive influences.

G. Aggressive behavior directed against people or property is less likely to recur if the teenager is supervised and treatment is less likely to be terminated impulsively if it is court mandated. Psychotherapy should help the patient understand the significance and consequences of his behavior. The family needs help to set limits on the child. Because of the high recidivism rate of aggressive behavior, if intense treatment of patient and family does not produce improvement within 6 months, residential treatment is necessary.

H. The poor prognosis of unsocialized patients indicates intensive treatment, and perhaps residential care. This care usually lasts 6 months to 2 years; the child then returns home. He is placed in another group living situation if antisocial behavior continues.

REFERENCES

Couger JJ. Adolescence and Youth. New York: Harper & Row, 1977.

Tooley K. The small assassins; clinical notes on a subgroup of murderous children. J Amer Acad Child Psychiatry 1975; 14:306–318.

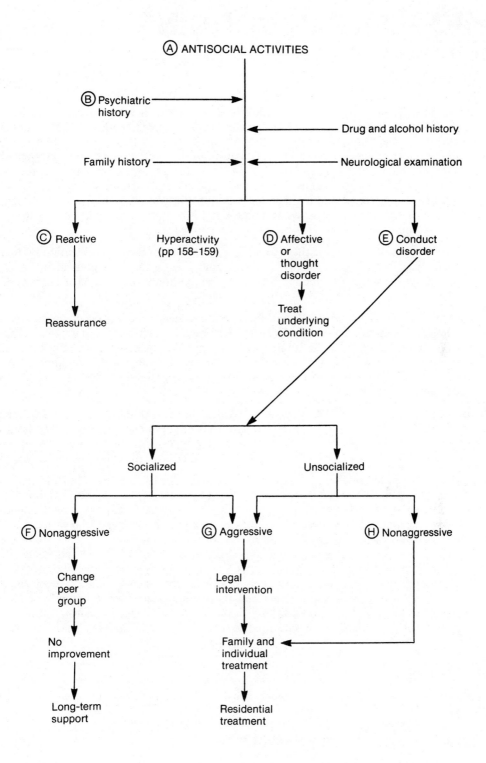

ANTISOCIAL ACTIVITIES

Psychiatric history

Drug and alcohol history

Family history

Neurological examination

Reactive

Hyperactivity (pp 158–159)

Affective or thought disorder

Conduct disorder

Reassurance

Treat underlying condition

Socialized

Unsocialized

Nonaggressive

Aggressive

Nonaggressive

Change peer group

Legal intervention

No improvement

Family and individual treatment

Long-term support

Residential treatment

Thomas A, Chess S, Birch HG. Temperament and Behavior Disorders in Children. New York: NYU Press, 1968.

PROBLEMS IN BONDING
William V. Good, M.D.

COMMENTS

A. Bonding is the process by which an emotional attachment develops between mother and child. Factors that warrant close observation of a pregnant woman for difficulty with bonding include: failure to obtain prenatal care; statements that the new child will be a burden or an intruder; other signs of extreme ambivalence about the pregnancy; pregnancy whose goal is to replace a lost loved one; pregnancy in an adolescent; maternal depression or psychosis; history of neglect or battering in either parent; marital discord, isolation, or lack of resources; overconcern about risk to the newborn; persistent overreaction to prenatally diagnosed fetal abnormality or neonatal illness or death of a previous child; and separation of infant and mother at birth.

B. Major psychiatric illness in either parent (e.g., postpartum depression) should be treated vigorously. If both parents express significant ambivalence about the pregnancy that is not resolved by discussion, the possibility of arranging adoption as soon after delivery as possible should be raised.

C. Since there is no critical period during which bonding does or does not occur, parents who do not bond immediately may gradually be able to form an attachment, even if it takes months. Signs of poor bonding include: failure to choose a name in the absence of cultural guidelines not to name immediately; avoidance of physical or eye contact with the infant; excessive protectiveness; derogatory statements about the infant; attribution of adult motivations to the infant; failure to thrive.

D. Bonding may be encouraged by regular physical contact with the child, or at least regular visits if the child cannot be touched. If a name has not been chosen, the parents should be encouraged to do so. The parents should be observed for evidence of realistic positive feelings toward, and a wish for emotional and physical contact with, the child.

E. If there is no good evidence of bonding, formal evaluation of parenting ability is necessary. Adoption, or at least immediate foster placement, is necessary if minimal bonding is associated with a high risk of abuse (pp 154–155), or emotional unresponsiveness or failure to thrive in the infant. Parents who do not present an immediate risk and who wish to keep the child may be observed in the hospital over a longer period of time. If bonding begins to develop, intensive outpatient follow-up is mandatory. Visiting nurses and pediatricians should monitor the infant's physical status; social service agencies should be contacted to provide appropriate support. Group therapy may decrease social isolation. Involvement of family members and other supports can help the parents to take care of the child and provide role models for parenting. Individual psychotherapy should focus on demonstrating appropriate infant care, which the parents are then asked to practice under supervision.

REFERENCES

Harmon R, Glickes A, Good W. A new book at maternal-infant bonding. Perinatol-Neonatol 1982; 9:27–31.

Klaus MH, Kennell JH. Parent-infant Bonding. St. Louis: CV Mosby, 1982.

Bowlby J. Attachment and Loss. New York: Basic Books, 1969.

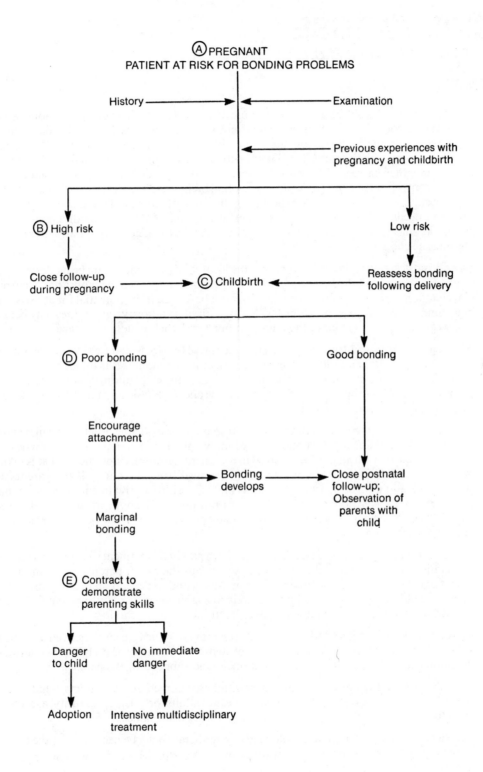

Ⓐ PREGNANT
PATIENT AT RISK FOR BONDING PROBLEMS

History ⟶ ⟵ Examination

⟵ Previous experiences with
pregnancy and childbirth

Ⓑ High risk　　　　　　　　　　　Low risk

Close follow-up　⟶ Ⓒ Childbirth ⟵ Reassess bonding
during pregnancy　　　　　　　following delivery

Ⓓ Poor bonding　　　　　　Good bonding

Encourage
attachment

Bonding ⟶ Close postnatal
develops　　follow-up;
Observation of
parents with
child

Marginal
bonding

Ⓔ Contract to
demonstrate
parenting skills

Danger　　　No immediate
to child　　　danger

Adoption　Intensive multidisciplinary
treatment

153

CHILD ABUSE
William V. Good, M.D.

COMMENTS

A. Child abuse includes physical and sexual abuse of any sort. The suspicion of child abuse arises from any accidental injury but especially repeated injuries; specific injuries likely to be purposeful; chronic multiple somatic complaints in a child; and complaints of parental inability to cope with the child. The potential for abuse is high if any one of the following are present in either parent: history of abuse as a child; psychosis; history of difficulty with impulse control; antisocial personality; perception of the child as older than he is; expectation that the child gratify the parents; expectation that the child carry out adult tasks; belief that the child needs frequent strong punishment; perception of the child as different or bad; emphatic, angry denial of the possibility of abuse. A relative, neighbor, or babysitter may be abusing the child.

B. Laws in most states require that a report to the local child protection team be made within 24 hours if parents or child admit abuse or if it is likely but not proven that abuse has occurred. Consultation with a child protection team should be sought if the potential for abuse seems high. Since many abusing parents are skilled at gratifying authority figures, they may behave like ideal caretakers in front of the physician but batter their children at home.

C. Abusing parents feel guilty and are extremely sensitive to criticism; the risk of abuse must be discussed openly but tactfully. Evaluation usually involves home visits by social workers or the police. Since the parents may conceal the danger to the child during home visits, a social agency should follow the high-risk family regularly, and the physician should remain alert for suspicious injuries and behavior.

D. If the danger is not high and sufficient social resources are available, treatment can begin in the home, thus minimizing disruption of the family unit. This decision should be made only after consultation with all parties involved in treatment. However, if physical abuse is taking place, the child's life may be saved by rapid removal from the home. If the parents are cooperative and can be trusted to follow through with the treatment plan, voluntary placement in a foster home may help them to feel positively about treatment; otherwise, involuntary placement is necessary and permanent placement must be considered if the danger remains high.

E. There should always be individual therapy for both parents. Treatment should focus on their expectations of the child and their relationships with their own parents. They should be taught to care for the child, to control their impulses, and to depend on the therapist rather than the child. Someone must be immediately available whenever either parent feels at all stressed to keep them from taking out their frustrations on the child.

F. Close supervision is required when the child remains in or returns to an abusive environment: regular home visits by social agencies, repeated evaluations of the child's psychosocial development, and ongoing psychiatric treatment and support for the parents.

G. Individual psychotherapy for the child, in addition to treatment for the parents, is indicated if the child demonstrates excessive compliance, fear of adults, precocious maturity, aggressive, seductive, or provocative behavior; or any psychiatric disturbance.

H. Even when the parents improve, prolonged psychotherapy may be necessary for the child in order to help him develop a realistic attitude toward his experiences, deal with his anger, and avoid abusing his own children.

REFERENCES

Kempe CH, Silverman FN, Steele BF, et al. The battered child syndrome. JAMA 1962; 181:17–20.
Kempe CH, Helfer R. The Battered Child. 2nd ed. Chicago: University of Chicago Press, 1974.

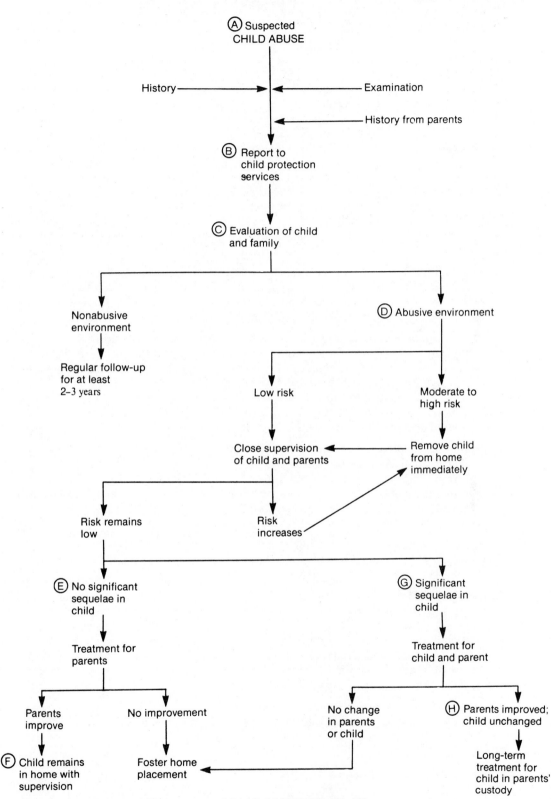

Ⓐ Suspected
CHILD ABUSE

History ⟶ ⟵ Examination

⟵ History from parents

Ⓑ Report to
child protection
services

Ⓒ Evaluation of child
and family

Nonabusive
environment

Regular follow-up
for at least
2–3 years

Ⓓ Abusive environment

Low risk

Moderate to
high risk

Close supervision
of child and parents ⟵ Remove child
from home
immediately

Risk remains
low

Risk
increases

Ⓔ No significant
sequelae in
child

Ⓖ Significant
sequelae in
child

Treatment for
parents

Treatment for
child and parent

Parents
improve

No improvement

No change
in parents
or child

Ⓗ Parents improved;
child unchanged

Ⓕ Child remains
in home with
supervision

Foster home
placement

Long-term
treatment for
child in parents'
custody

Jaffe AC. Sexual abuse of children. Amer J Dis Child 1975; 129:689–692.

CHILDHOOD DEPRESSION
William V. Good, M.D.

COMMENTS

A. Anaclitic depression in infancy (age 7–30 mos) is diagnosed according to criteria on page 168. Little is known about the incidence, diagnosis, and treatment of depression in children aged 30 mos–6 yrs. From late childhood to adolescence, depression presents with the following symptoms: depressed mood; social withdrawal, loss of interest in usual activities; feelings of helplessness; difficulties in school; conduct disturbances (pp 150–151), substance abuse; atypical symptoms such as overeating, hypersomnia, or extreme fatigue. A positive dexamethasone suppression test (utilizing 0.5 instead of 1 mg of dexamethasone) is highly correlated (60–70%) with a diagnosis of endogenous depression. Medical illnesses that are particularly likely to produce depression in children include hyper- and hypothyroidism, Addison's disease, Wilson's disease, porphyria, and drug ingestion, withdrawal (especially amphetamines), or side effects (especially of drugs used to treat childhood hypertension such as reserpine and methyldopa).

B. Depression in children may occur in reaction to a problem in the family, especially if it threatens him with separation from an important caretaker. Children with a family history of depression, suicide, mania, alcoholism, and antisocial behavior are vulnerable to depression. Family therapy is necessary to resolve problems that the family avoids confronting.

C. Children experience the same symptoms of grief as adults, although behavioral disturbances, especially agitation and withdrawal, are more prominent. Prolonged disturbed behavior, refusal to talk about the loss, absence of overt signs of grief, psychosomatic symptoms, vegetative signs, guilt, and lowered self-esteem indicate that grief is not being expressed normally and is evolving into depression. Frequently the parents are not helping the child to grieve. Open mourning should be encouraged in all children who have sustained a loss; the family should be helped to share the child's grief.

D. Depression in children can be caused by problems in negotiating normal developmental tasks. These problems may be caused by: prolonged early separation from a primary caretaker; prolonged illness or parental unwillingness to allow independence; harsh treatment by the parent of the same sex or rejection by the parent of the opposite sex; and inability to form relationships outside the family. Specific treatment is aimed at minimizing these difficulties.

E. When a child's depression occurs in imitation of a depressed adult, the adult should be treated first. Treatment for the child is indicated if the child does not improve following the adult's recovery.

F. If individual treatment is unsuccessful, the family should be involved more intensively; if family therapy has been the primary modality, the patient should be seen separately. Antidepressants may be of definite help to some pediatric patients. The usual dose is 1.5 mg/kg/day of imipramine in 3 divided doses. Under no circumstances should a dose of 4.5 mg/kg/day be exceeded. Childproof packaging is essential. Failure to improve within 4–6 months indicates the more intensive therapy in a residential center for 6 months to 3 years, along with treatment of family pathological adaptations.

G. Little is known about factors associated with risk of relapse; indefinite follow-up once or twice a year is indicated to monitor for reemergence of symptoms at times of similar stress.

REFERENCES

Puig-Antich J. Major depression and conduct disorder in prepuberty. J Amer Acad Child Psychiatry 1982; 21:118–128.

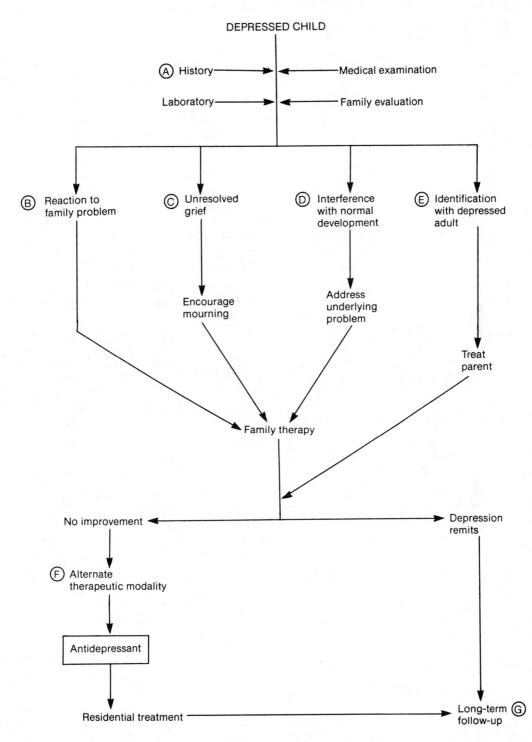

Kashami JH. Current perspectives on childhood depression: an overview. Amer J Psychiatry 1981; 138:143–147.
Cytryn L, McKnew D. Affective disorders. In: Kaplan HI, Freedman AM, Sadock BJ. Comprehensive Textbook of Psychiatry. 3rd ed. Baltimore: Williams & Wilkins, 1980: 2798–2810.

BEHAVIOR PROBLEMS IN SCHOOL

William V. Good, M.D.

COMMENTS

A. Behavioral disturbances in school have a wide range of causes and severity. The first step is to ascertain the timing and extent of the problem. Misbehavior in only one class may indicate a conflict with a particular student or teacher, while intermittent disturbances may represent the child's reaction to family conflicts. Evaluation of conflicts and examination for covert encouragement of behavior problems by the family is essential. Behavioral changes that emerge at school may be caused by a developing psychosis or by a number of physical illnesses, including degenerative diseases, temporal lobe epilepsy, endocrine disorders, vitamin deficiencies, and lead poisoning. Early involvement of school authorities elicits important information and helps implement the treatment plan. Teachers should be encouraged to ask the child about his feelings, not to reward disruptive behavior with increased attention, and to exclude the child from class if he cannot control his behavior.

B. Fear of going to school (pp 164–165) is usually due to separation anxiety, often shared by the parents. School phobia, or hyperactivity that is only present at school, may also be a reaction to a specific situation or classroom topic that frightens the patient or arouses unresolved conflicts, often concerning sex or aggression. Some stresses, such as exposure to an antagonistic fellow student, can reasonably be changed. If the child is afraid of a situation that cannot or should not be changed, such as showering with other students or learning about sex, psychotherapy may help the child control his concerns. If insight alone does not resolve situational hyperactivity, a stimulant such as methylphenidate (5–40 mg/day in divided doses) may be administered on school days. Behavioral disturbances caused by the frustration of a child with a learning disorder usually abate when a remedial program is instituted.

C. Disturbed behavior in response to a crisis abates with treatment of the underlying problem, as do behavioral disturbances that are symptomatic of major depression, mania, or schizophrenia.

D. Hyperactivity is a syndrome of exaggerated motor activity, decreased attention span, and impulsivity. Attention deficit disorder is not associated with any signs of brain dysfunction; psychological and constitutional factors are presumed to be causative. If psychotherapy and family therapy do not control the patient's behavior, stimulants may be helpful. Distractability and hyperactivity may continue into adult life, when signs of personality disorder may begin to appear.

E. Gross brain dysfunction may be associated with hyperactivity that can be controlled by assigning concrete tasks that the child can accomplish, rewarding constructive behavior, and ignoring or punishing disruptive behavior. If hyperactivity is a paradoxical reaction to sedating medications, the dosage should be reduced or the drug changed.

REFERENCES

Lassers E, Mordan R, Blackholm S. Steps in the return to school of children with school problems. Amer J Psychiatry 1973; 130:265–270.

Schmidt BD. The hyperactive child. Clin Pediat 1973; 12:154–169.

Walraich ML. Stimulant drug therapy in hyperactive children. Pediatrics 1977; 60:512–518.

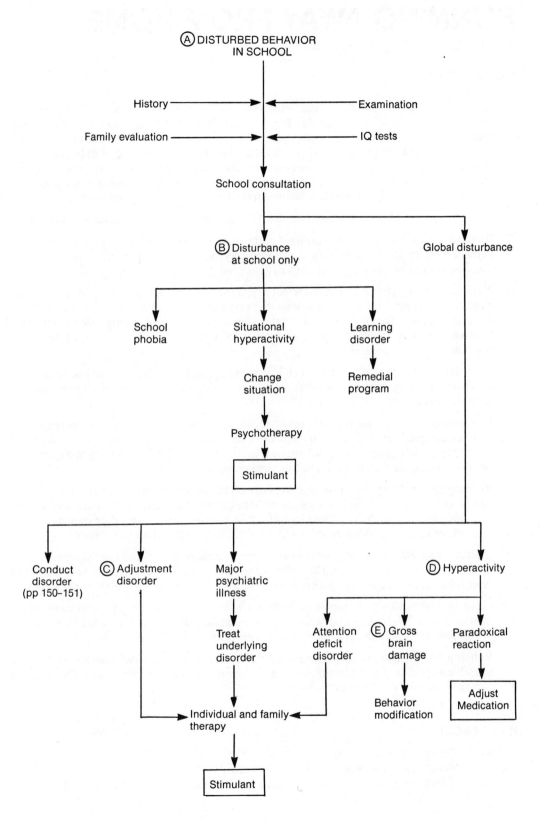

(A) DISTURBED BEHAVIOR
IN SCHOOL

History ──────────► ◄────────── Examination

Family evaluation ──────────► ◄────────── IQ tests

School consultation

(B) Disturbance
at school only

Global disturbance

School
phobia

Situational
hyperactivity

Learning
disorder

Change
situation

Remedial
program

Psychotherapy

Stimulant

Conduct
disorder
(pp 150–151)

(C) Adjustment
disorder

Major
psychiatric
illness

(D) Hyperactivity

Treat
underlying
disorder

Attention
deficit
disorder

(E) Gross
brain
damage

Paradoxical
reaction

Individual and family
therapy

Behavior
modification

Adjust
Medication

Stimulant

RUNNING AWAY FROM HOME

William V. Good, M.D.

COMMENTS

A. Running away is second only to drug abuse among childhood behavioral problems. Between 600,000 and 1 million American children run away from home each year. If threats to run away have been present for some time, the behavior likely reflects a deeply entrenched means of handling family conflicts. Running away may represent the child's attempt to free himself from a family that cannot tolerate separation. Other indication of difficulty in establishing independence include school phobia, few friends, staying too close to home, or staying away from home excessively. Incest may be involved when adolescent girls run away.

B. The child is more likely to return to the family if they are willing to understand his behavior.

C. Runaways should be reported to the local authorities. Friends may also be able to help and to negotiate his return. If these efforts are unsuccessful, national agencies, may be helpful. Grieving should be encouraged if runaway children do not return.

D. The parents should be advised not to react angrily or make inappropriate promises when the child contacts them or returns. Problems that may have arisen during his absence should be discussed openly. The physician must help the parents to express strong reactions to these problems without conveying excessive blame; the child should be encouraged to air his reactions to his experiences.

E. Brain damaged or mentally retarded children may wander away from home and forget how to return. If sufficient constant supervision cannot be provided by the family, day care or institutional care may be necessary.

F. Psychotic children are particularly prone to run away as a means of separating from their families. Hospitalization is necessary to control the patient and institute intensive treatment if severe psychopathology is not resolving or if the patient repeatedly runs away and engages in behavior that is dangerous to himself or someone else.

G. Running away may occur in anticipation of punishment or criticism or in reaction to a family, school, or social crisis. Four to six visits should be devoted to discussing the crisis and helping the family to reassure the child that he will not be punished excessively if he returns. Family conflicts of longer standing must be addressed if the behavior does not resolve.

H. Children who are talked into running away by their peers usually are overly dependent on others for nurturing or identity. They often return when they find that the peer group does not meet their needs adequately. Intensive discussion of these insecurities may be necessary.

I. Children who run away whenever they are upset are likely to run away from any outpatient treatment that fails to make them feel good immediately. Residential treatment is necessary to control their behavior long enough for them to look into their conflicts.

J. Running away usually occurs because the family has been unable to teach the child more adaptive ways of dealing with conflict. Family therapy is essential to address conflicts that are avoided when the child leaves the family.

REFERENCES

Jenkins RL. The runaway reaction. Amer J Psychiatry 1971; 128:163–173.

Raphael M, Wolf J. Runaways. New York: Drake Publishers, 1974.

Stierles H. A family perspective on adolescent runaways. Arch Gen Psychiatry 1973; 29:56–62.

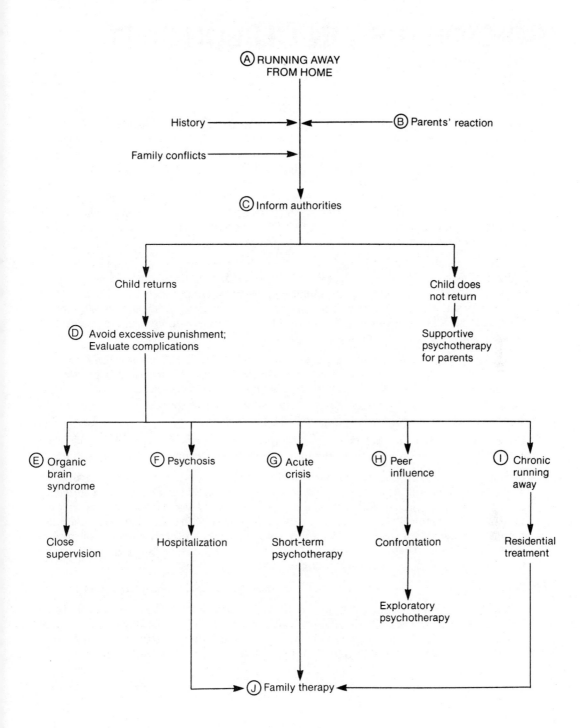

A RUNNING AWAY FROM HOME

History ⟶ ⟵ B Parents' reaction

Family conflicts ⟶

C Inform authorities

Child returns

Child does not return

D Avoid excessive punishment; Evaluate complications

Supportive psychotherapy for parents

E Organic brain syndrome

F Psychosis

G Acute crisis

H Peer influence

I Chronic running away

Close supervision

Hospitalization

Short-term psychotherapy

Confrontation

Residential treatment

Exploratory psychotherapy

J Family therapy

SUICIDE RISK IN CHILDHOOD
William V. Good, M.D.

COMMENTS

A. Depressed, withdrawn, and schizophrenic children are at high risk for suicide and should be evaluated routinely for suicide risk. The incidence of suicide in children under the age of 14 appears to be increasing. Suicide risk in childhood is increased by: unresolved grief over a lost family member; depression and suicidal behavior in parents; accident proneness; poor impulse control; access to potential means of suicide; belief that death is pleasant, not permanent, or can be undone by wishing (such magical thoughts dominate thinking under age 4 or 5 and may persist until age 10–11); and chronic illness, drug abuse, or psychosis. The child may not understand the word "suicide"; other expressions such as "make yourself die" may have to be found.

B. Psychotherapy should attempt to elucidate the child's vulnerability to certain events. Episodic self-destructive behavior is especially likely to emerge in the following circumstances: (1) a disciplinary crisis: one-third of childhood suicide attempts occur in anticipation of disciplinary action; (2) separation from a parent: the child experiences the parent's absence as the parent's death and wants to join the parent; (3) rejection or severe embarassment; and (4) a birthday, for unknown reasons.

C. Severely depressed or schizophrenic children who suffer from extremely low self-esteem or pessimism may have a pervasive wish to die. Suicidal impulses increase as depression or psychosis deepens. Some psychotic children injure themselves to experience a strong physical sensation, not to die. Major depression in children often responds to antidepressants. Schizophrenic children should receive a trial of neuroleptics.

D. Children may learn to manipulate their parents by threatening suicide. Some of these children are frightened of being alone; they attempt suicide to coerce people into staying with them.

E. Because children do not have the cognitive ability to calculate a nonlethal attempt accurately, any child who threatens or attempts suicide should be hospitalized and watched closely to evaluate the seriousness of the problem. The patient needs help to improve interpersonal skills and self-esteem and find alternative methods of coping with suicidal ideation. Families should be evaluated for violence, incest, rejection of the child, or covert sanctions of suicidal behavior. Additional help may be sought from self-help groups such as Systematic Training for Effective Parenting or National Alliance for the Mentally Ill.

F. Successful return to school after a suicide attempt is a particularly favorable prognostic sign.

G. If suicidal ideation does not remit quickly, inpatient treatment for months is likely to be necessary to control the child's behavior. Continued risk of suicide is likely to be related to serious chronic psychopathology in the family. Alternative living situations may help until pathological interactions can be treated. If this fails, long-term residential care is necessary.

REFERENCES

Roy A. Family history of suicide. Arch Gen Psychiatry 1983; 40:971–978.
Kashani JH, Husain A, Shekim WO, et al. Current perspectives on childhood depression: an overview. Am J Psychiatry 1981; 138:145–153.
Wiener JM. Psychopharmacology in Children and Adolescence. New York: Basic Book, 1977.
Orbach I, Glaubman H. The concept of death and suicidal behavior in young children. J Amer Acad Child Psychiatry 1979; 18:668–678.
Pfeffer CR. Suicidal behavior of children: a review with implications for research and practice. Amer J Psychiatry 1981; 138:154–159.

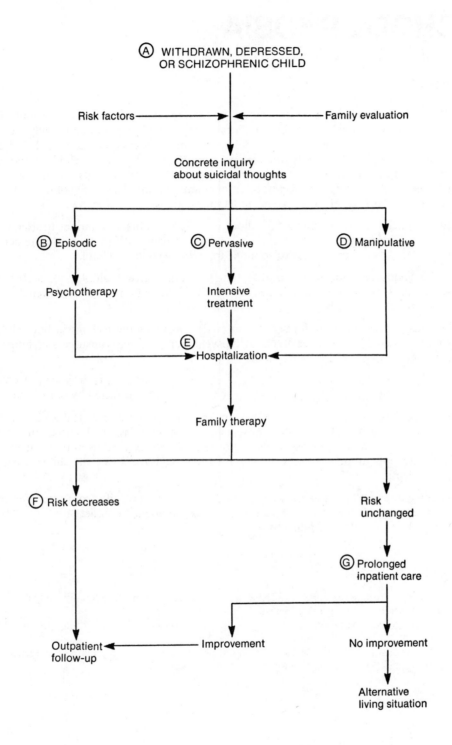

(A) WITHDRAWN, DEPRESSED,
OR SCHIZOPHRENIC CHILD

Risk factors ———————→ ←——————— Family evaluation

Concrete inquiry
about suicidal thoughts

(B) Episodic   (C) Pervasive   (D) Manipulative

Psychotherapy   Intensive
                     treatment

(E) Hospitalization

Family therapy

(F) Risk decreases   Risk
                                      unchanged

                                      (G) Prolonged
                                          inpatient care

Outpatient ←——————— Improvement   No improvement
follow-up

                                       Alternative
                                       living situation

Morrison GC. Emergencies in Child Psychiatry: Emotional Crises of Youth and Their Families. Springfield,
    Illinois: CC Thomas, 1975.

163

SCHOOL PHOBIA
William V. Good, M.D.

COMMENTS

A. School phobia usually manifests as outright refusal to attend school. Less frequently, it may be disguised as stomach aches, feigned illness, and accident proneness, especially if the child without documented illness misses school more than 3 times in 6 weeks. School phobia may begin at any age. It is usually due to separation anxiety in younger children and fear of exposure of their bodies or in rare instances, psychosis, in adolescents. Conflict with other students or abusive teachers may be additional motivations. The family of the patient with separation anxiety often covertly encourages the child to stay home.

B. Even if the child is very frightened of school, it is important that he continue to attend so that avoidance does not become habitual and the patient can learn to master his anxiety. The parents need to be encouraged to continue to send the child to school.

C. If school phobia is associated with additional symptoms such as multiple phobias, behavioral disturbances, or hyperactivity, thorough psychiatric evaluation is indicated even if the child returns to school rapidly.

D. Short-term psychotherapy for separation anxiety explores the feelings in both child and parents that lead to avoidance of school. If psychotherapy alone is unsuccessful, imipramine may alleviate early onset school phobia.

E. Change to another school may be necessary if documented threats or violence from other students or unnecessary humiliation by teachers cannot be corrected by school authorities.

F. Young adolescents may be afraid of exposing their bodies during physical education classes because of shyness, fears of being homosexual, or self-consciousness. If reassurance does not help the patient return to classes, he may be temporarily excused from physical education while attending all other classes. Psychotherapy should investigate the child's anxieties in greater depth.

G. Inability to complete assigned work should not excuse the child from attending school. Educational problems require tutoring, while psychological conflicts that interfere with learning must be addressed directly.

REFERENCES

Rodriguez A, Rodriguez M, Eisenberg L. The outcome of school phobia: a follow-up study based on 41 cases. Amer J Psychiatry 1959; 116:540–543.

Malinquist CP. School phobia: a problem in family neurosis. J Amer Acad Child Psychiatry 1965; 4:293–299.

Farley GK, Eckhardt LO, Hebert FB. Handbook of Child and Adolescent Psychiatric Emergencies. New York: Medical Examination Publishing, 1976: 102–112.

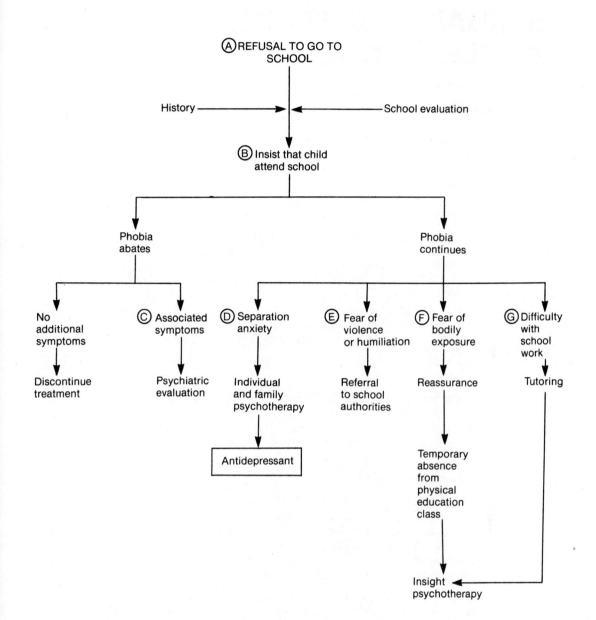

Ⓐ REFUSAL TO GO TO SCHOOL

History ⟶ ⟵ School evaluation

Ⓑ Insist that child attend school

Phobia abates

Phobia continues

No additional symptoms

Ⓒ Associated symptoms

Ⓓ Separation anxiety

Ⓔ Fear of violence or humiliation

Ⓕ Fear of bodily exposure

Ⓖ Difficulty with school work

Discontinue treatment

Psychiatric evaluation

Individual and family psychotherapy

Referral to school authorities

Reassurance

Tutoring

Antidepressant

Temporary absence from physical education class

Insight psychotherapy

SEXUAL ACTIVITY IN ADOLESCENCE

William V. Good, M.D.

COMMENTS

A. Curiosity about differences between the sexes and about parental sexuality and sexual activity in the form of kissing and masturbation normally begin by age 3–5 years. Before age 5, sexual behavior may be direct, or it may be displaced in the form of playing with dolls. Sexual expression through "playing doctor" and similar games is common in latency age (5–12 yrs) children; the range of sexual activity that occurs during adolescence depends to a great extent on family values, peer group and rebellion against the family.

B. Adolescents who are given insufficient information and support by their families can benefit greatly from education by the physician. Adolescents will forego birth control but not intercourse if parental permission is required. Most girls become pregnant within 6 months of initial intercourse if they do not use birth control. Recent court rulings have upheld the physician's right to counsel and prescribe birth control to adolescents without notifying the parents. The psychological and physical risks of teenage motherhood are greater than those of abortion; teenage marriages are at higher risk, especially when occasioned by a pregnancy, as are subsequent marriages in women who were first married as teenagers.

C. Promiscuous sexual behavior is abnormal. It may be an expression of depression, difficulty separating from parents, covert psychosis, or personality disorder.

D. Many transvestites are heterosexual; others dress in women's clothing to make their homosexuality more acceptable by assuring a feminine role. Over time, homosexual interest may increase even in the former group. Transvestism (pp 128–129) has only been reported in boys and men; it may appear in childhood. Intensive psychotherapy may be helpful.

E. Homosexual experimentation in early adolescence is common and normal. The physician should see the patient once every year or two to monitor development of sexual preference.

F. From 10 to 15% of the population is primarily homosexual (pp 120–121). Sexual identity and preference probably develop in early childhood; few people change sexual preference once it has been firmly established. Complaints by an adolescent about homosexual preference often reflect his or the family's discomfort. Helping the patient adjust to his sexual choice, educating the family, and healing ruptures in family relationships are indicated in such situations, as is a supportive, nonjudgmental attitude. Self-help groups may be appropriate.

G. Transsexualism, which occurs only in males, consists of an inner conviction of being a member of the opposite sex, effeminate mannerisms, transvestism, and a wish to associate with children of the opposite sex. This disorder usually begins to develop by 2 years of age, often in the youngest sibling, in a child who is abnormally close to a mother who has an intense dislike of men and a father who is emotionally distant or unavailable. Schizophrenia, depression, and homosexuality can all be associated with requests for sex change. The transvestite has a masculine identity and does not wish to change his sex.

H. Every attempt should be made to alter disturbances of gender identity discovered in childhood. The family should be involved in all phases of treatment. By adolescence, it becomes difficult, if not impossible, to change gender identity. After prolonged intensive treatment, sex change surgery may need to be considered.

REFERENCES

Green R. Gender identity disorders of childhood. In: Kaplan HI, Freedman AM, Sadock BJ, eds. Comprehensive Textbook of Psychiatry. 3rd ed. Baltimore: Williams & Wilkins, 1980: 2774–2781.

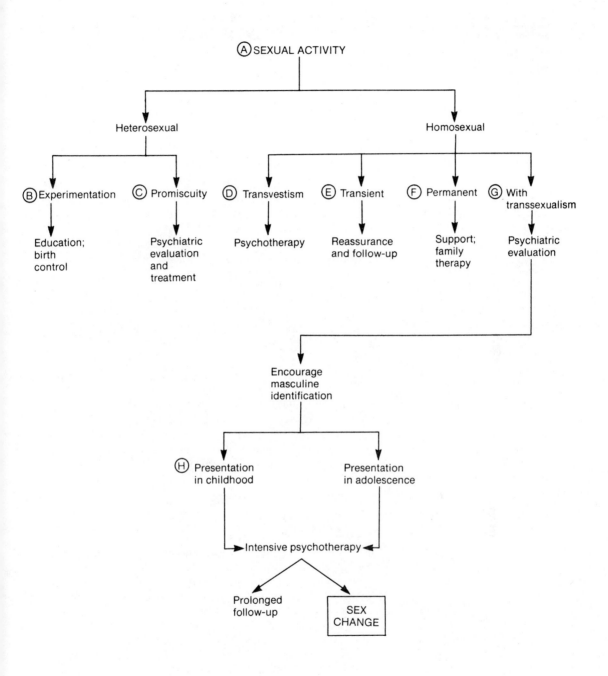

Ⓐ SEXUAL ACTIVITY

Heterosexual

Ⓑ Experimentation   Ⓒ Promiscuity

Education;
birth
control

Psychiatric
evaluation
and
treatment

Homosexual

Ⓓ Transvestism   Ⓔ Transient   Ⓕ Permanent   Ⓖ With
transsexualism

Psychotherapy   Reassurance
and follow-up   Support;
family
therapy   Psychiatric
evaluation

Encourage
masculine
identification

Ⓗ Presentation
in childhood   Presentation
in adolescence

Intensive psychotherapy

Prolonged
follow-up   SEX
CHANGE

Stoller RJ. Sex and Gender. New York: Science House, 1968.
Green R, Money J. Transsexualism and Sex Reassignment. Baltimore: Johns Hopkins University Press,
    1969.

SOCIAL UNRESPONSIVENESS IN CHILDREN

William V. Good, M.D.

COMMENTS

A. Social withdrawal in children may be caused by dehydration, meningitis, encephalitis, end-stage liver disease, metabolic disorders, congenital infections, and mental retardation.

B. Infants 6–30 months of age whose parents are physically or emotionally unavailable for prolonged periods of time may develop anaclitic depression (marasmus), characterized by withdrawal, unresponsiveness, sad faces, anorexia, and failure to thrive. Even if physical caretaking is good, the infant may die if insufficient emotional nurturing is provided. Visits to hospitalized children should be unrestricted to prevent separation reactions. Children with anaclitic depression whose parents are unavailable must be provided a consistent surrogate caretaker.

C. Treatment begins with a thoroughly reliable, stable, supportive, therapeutic relationship. Psychotherapy to help master overwhelming feelings of loss is possible once the child can communicate symbolically through play (age 20–24 mos). Long-term follow-up is necessary; children who have had anaclitic depression are predisposed to depressive symptoms if they experience later separations.

D. Retarded children with global developmental delays may seem autistic; 70% of autistic children have IQs <70. Retardation is more frequent in lower socioeconomic strata and results in consistently poor performance on all IQ tests and globally delayed speech development. Autism, which occurs in all socioeconomic classes, is associated with inconsistent IQ performance, with high scores on some subtests. Characteristic peculiarities of speech include echolalia, pronoun reversal, and slips of the tongue. Unlike some retardation syndromes, autism is not familial. If the diagnosis is unclear, a trial of treatment for autism, which has a somewhat better prognosis, is indicated.

E. Impaired hearing, which is commonly caused by hyperbilirubinemia, meningitis, encephalitis, and congenital defects may underly social unresponsiveness. If audiometry is inconclusive, auditory evoked potentials may reveal disturbances in auditory pathways.

F. When organic factors cannot be identified, infantile autism (Kanner's syndrome) and pervasive developmental disorder are likely causes of severe social unresponsiveness in children. Autism usually develops in early infancy, and always by age 30 months. Signs or symptoms include diminished or absent social responsiveness, abnormal response to the environment (stereotyped movements; obsessive need for sameness), and abnormalities of language. Pervasive developmental disorder appears after age 30 months and is similar to but less severe than autism, probably because the genetic load is less profound. Signs and symptoms include impaired socialization, clinging, lack of empathy for others, episodic intense anxiety, stereotyped movements, oddities of speech, and self-mutilating and aggressive behavior. Children with autism and pervasive developmental disorder need to be taught social skills in a highly structured environment. Behavior modification may help to motivate the patient to participate in educational and social activities. Medications (e.g., thioridazine 10–25 mg per day) are useful only for severe agitation. The parents need psychotherapy to help them deal with frustration and guilt, and advice about how to teach the child to interact. From 70 to 90% of these children never function outside the family or an institution, and many develop major motor seizures before adolescence. In the rest, affect and interpersonal skills are restricted.

SOCIALLY UNRESPONSIVE INFANT

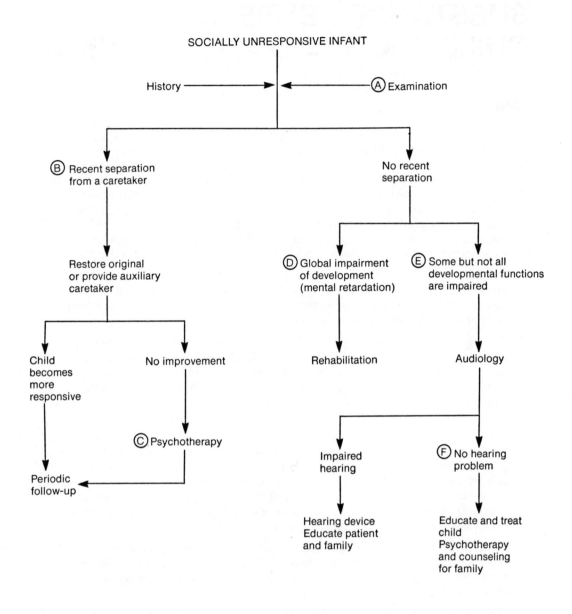

REFERENCES

Miller RT. Childhood schizophrenia: a review of selected literature. Internat J Ment Health 1973; 3:3–46.
Farley G, Eckhardt L, Hebert FB. Handbook of Child and Adolescent Psychiatric Emergencies. New York: Medical Examination Publishing, 1979.
Ritvo E. Autism: Diagnosis, Current Research and Management. New York: Spectrum Publications, 1976.

SUBSTANCE ABUSE IN CHILDHOOD AND ADOLESCENCE

William V. Good, M.D.

COMMENTS

A. Substance abuse occurs at least experimentally in 60–90% of all children and adolescents and has been reported in children as young as age 5. Drug or alcohol abuse in children and adolescents may present as accidents, intoxication (children may exhibit paradoxical sedation with amphetamines and hyperactivity with sedatives), abstinence syndromes (pp 112–113), poor school performance, social withdrawal, or personality change. Stigmata of parenteral abuse (e.g., needle tracks) and physical evidence of intoxication or withdrawal confirm the diagnosis. The patient should be asked directly which drugs are being abused, the extent of abuse, and the influence of friends. Motivation to deal with drug abuse is indicated by willingness to admit a problem, requests for help, and ability to tolerate drug-free periods.

B. Adolescents may experiment with a variety of drugs, often in a social setting, because of peer pressure and curiosity about the drug's effect. Alcohol and marijuana are commonly used experimentally by normal children; they should be counseled about possible adverse affects and followed for 6 months to ensure that abuse does not develop.

C. Patients experiencing family disruption, school problems, athletic or social failures, or other disappointments may experiment with drugs to relieve anxiety. An attempt should first be made to resolve the environmental stress. If the stress cannot be resolved, the patient and his family may need to examine the problem more intensively and find more constructive ways of adapting to it.

D. Chronic drug abuse has as its goal the experience of drug effects rather than experimentation or relief of anxiety and does not always occur in a social setting. Because of the likelihood of continued drug use and the danger of abstinence syndromes, inpatient detoxification is preferred for ongoing abuse. If the patient refuses detoxification, he may still be treated if his parents agree. If the parents refuse treatment, the physician should remain available. If substance abuse poses a threat to the patient's or someone else's life, involuntary inpatient treatment may be ordered by the physician even if the parents are uncooperative (pp 142–143). Legal consultation is necessary under such complicated circumstances.

E. Schizophrenic and depressed children may attempt to treat themselves with illicit drugs. Since intoxication and withdrawal from many substances, especially amphetamines, may mimic schizophrenia and depression, observation in a drug-free state is necessary to diagnose the underlying illness.

F. Since 70–80% of drug abusing patients with personality disorders relapse after detoxification, a prolonged inpatient program is necessary to prevent further drug abuse and begin psychotherapy to help the patient understand his motivations. Before discharge, an attempt should be made to change the patient's peer group if it is a bad influence, decrease his access to drugs, treat family problems, and arrange for close outpatient supervision. Periodic unscheduled urine screens can be used to assess compliance.

REFERENCES

Brecker EM. Licit and Illicit Drugs. Boston: Little, Brown, 1972.

Grinspoon L, Bakalar J. Drug dependence. In: Kaplan HI, Freedman AM, Sadock BJ, eds. Comprehensive Textbook of Psychiatry. 3rd ed. Baltimore: Williams & Wilkins, 1980: 1614–1629.

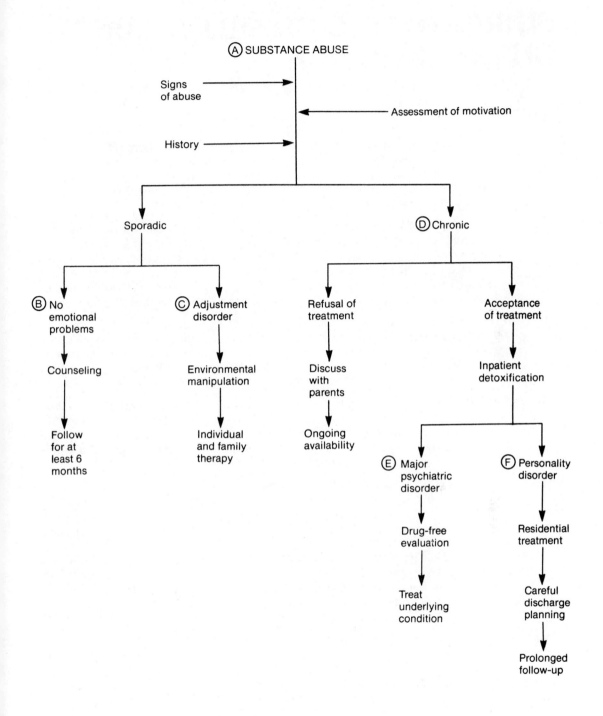

THREATS TO SIGN OUT AGAINST MEDICAL ADVICE

Troy L. Thompson, II, M.D. and Michael G. Moran, M.D.

COMMENTS

A. Patients usually threaten to leave the hospital after escalating confrontations with the medical staff. Investigate past episodes of refusal of treatment and their outcome, understanding of fears related to the illness and therapy, and presence of a mental disorder in case involuntary treatment is required or requested. Family members and other supports can be extremely helpful in securing temporary compliance.

B. Patients with organic brain syndromes may wish to leave the hospital because they are confused and frightened. Using concrete terms, remind the patient where he is and why he needs treatment. A strong suggestion that the patient remain in the hospital may help him to continue treatment until the impulse to leave, which is usually transient, passes. Unrestricted visits by familiar people and frequent checks by nursing staff decrease agitation. Low-dose nonsedating neuroleptics may decrease anxiety if other measures are unsuccessful.

C. Anxiety about the illness usually results in threats to leave the hospital if the patient's principle means of dealing with anxiety has been denial and the denial has broken down. Support of repression of anxiety with anxiolytics and reassurance may restore equilibrium, especially if the physician remains calm and does not increase the patient's anxiety by threatening dire consequences if the patient leaves.

D. Patients who feel they are being ignored or mistreated may call attention to their disappointment and anger by complaining about their care. If these complaints are not acknowledged, they may then escalate to threats to leave the hospital. Realistic complaints should be heeded and the patient's sensitivities approached respectfully. Minor concessions such as allowing the patient a special privilege may reassure him that he is being taken seriously.

E. Escalating power struggles usually result in the patient's proving that he, not the physician is in control by leaving the hospital. If the illness is resolving and the patient has simply set his own discharge date, he should be allowed to leave with as positive a feeling as possible about the physician and the treatment in order to maximize later compliance. If further hospital treatment is definitely necessary, a brief pass may help the patient to agree to further treatment. Involuntary treatment (pp 142–143) may be necessary if the patient's life is in immediate danger or a mental disorder is present. If the patient cannot be kept in the hospital, the physician should attempt to remain in contact with the patient and the family to facilitate later return to the hospital.

REFERENCES

Albert HO, Kornfeld DS. The threat to sign out against medical advice. Ann Intern Med 1973; 79–888.

Hackett TP. Disruptive states. In: Hackett TP, Carsen NH, eds. Massachusetts General Hospital Handbook of General Hospital Psychiatry. St. Louis: CV Mosby, 1978: 231.

Jankowski CB, Drum DE. Diagnostic correlates of discharge against medical advice. Arch Gen Psychiatry 1977; 34:153.

Schlauch RW, Reich P, Kelly MJ. Leaving the hospital against medical advice. N Engl J Med 1979; 300: 22.

Tupin JP. Management of violent patients. In: Shader RI, ed. Manual of Psychiatric Therapeutics. Boston: Little Brown, 1976.

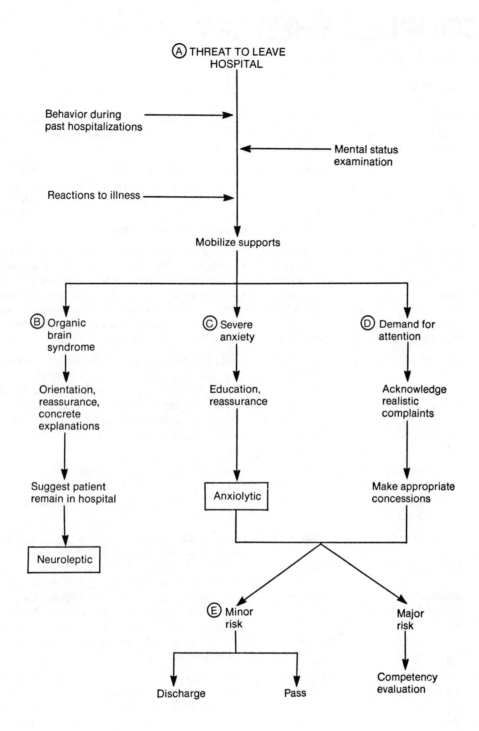

COUPLES THERAPY

Steven L. Dubovsky, M.D.

COMMENTS

A. Whenever a couple complains of a problem in the relationship or a patient describes a complaint that involves a partner, an attempt should be made to direct treatment toward the couple in addition to or instead of toward either individual.

B. Initial history includes how the couple met, relationship with families of origin and with children, psychiatric treatment of either partner, the partners' expectations of each other and of treatment, sexual functioning, financial problems, ability of each partner to be alone, and patterns of communication. Although it may initially seem time consuming, involving the partner actually saves time because the real problems are addressed.

C. Statements by the presenting patient that the partner refuses to be involved in couples (conjoint) therapy may reflect a covert wish to have the therapist's undivided attention or to avoid confronting painful problems in the relationship. Treatment should focus on these concerns and on ways of encouraging the partner to participate. If the partner continues to refuse therapy, the patient's reasons for continuing an unsatisfactory relationship should be addressed. Self-help groups for spouses of patients with special problems may offer necessary support if the presenting patient refuses to consider separation.

D. A request for help with irreconcilable marital problems may mask a wish that the therapist will suggest separation or that difficulties can magically be resolved. The couple may also seek alleviation of fears of separation. Discussion of feelings about independence, finances, dating, and care of the children minimizes later bitterness; education that divorce is less harmful to children than prolonged bitter marriage may also allay a common concern. If the couple decides to separate, they should be helped to grieve the loss of a relationship they once valued.

E. If, when it is pointed out by the therapist, the couple does not stop destructive interactions, the interaction should be interrupted. Each partner may then be asked to state his or her position. Asking one partner to imagine the other's point of view may reveal distortions in their perceptions of each other.

F. People may enter relationships with expectations that they may not convey openly to the other person because of a fear of rejection or because they are consciously unaware of them. Common expectations include unconditional love, caretaking or support, financial security, control of the other person, and compensation for past hardships. Disappointment and anger because of unfulfilled expectations may not become apparent until they are clarified in psychotherapy. When one partner expects to save the other from a severe psychiatric, personality, or even criminal disorder in order to meet his or her own grandiose or masochistic needs, helping both partners to recognize the seriousness of the patient's problem is a necessary step in reorganizing the couple's relationship.

G. Clarification involves stating unspoken expectations and reactions explicitly and pointing out ways in which the partners compete with each other for attention, nurturing, and power. Marital discord frequently results from failure to communicate needs and feelings openly. When specific difficulties are uncovered, disruptive habits may be altered by behavioral assignments.

H. When one partner is found to have a psychiatric disorder that is reflected in disturbances in addition to discord in the relationship, individual psychological and pharmacological treatment may be added to, but should not replace, conjoint therapy.

I. Other members of the immediate or extended family may encourage problems in the relationship, or one partner may feel that a commitment to the relationship is disloyal to

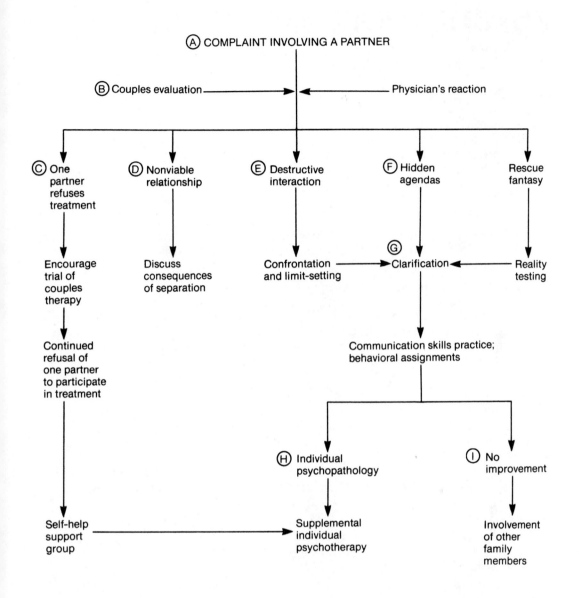

someone else in the family. When these problems arise, therapy may need to involve other family members.

REFERENCES

Berman E. The treatment of troubled couples. In: Grinspoon L, ed. Psychiatry Update, Vol. II. Washington, DC: APA Press, 1982: 215–228.

Berman EM, Lief HI. Marital therapy from a psychiatric perspective. Amer J Psychiatry 1975; 132:583–592.

Jacobson N, Margolin G. Marital Therapy. New York: Brunner/Mazel, 1979.

PSYCHOLOGICAL TESTING

Eugene P. Schwartz, Ph.D.,
Gregory Steinwand, Psy.D.

COMMENTS

A. Psychological testing often provides information that the patient is unable or unwilling to discuss openly. Data obtained are objective and empirically based and not biased by countertransference or other reactions evoked by an ongoing relationship with the patient. A broad battery of tests includes *objective* tests such as the WAIS, *empirical* tests such as the MMPI, and *projective* tests such as the Rorshach and TAT. The psychologist selects specific tests best suited to the clinical situation. Most tests can detect conscious and unconscious attempts to exaggerate or conceal inner distress.

B. Baseline data to be obtained prior to testing include history of the present illness, description of psychotic symptoms, premorbid level of functioning, mental status examination, and circumstances such as legal problems surrounding the evaluation.

C. Interest tests such as the Strong Vocational Interest Blank and ability tests measuring such areas as mechanical and cognitive aptitude may assist in career planning or reassessment of current job choice. Psychological testing can help clarify equivocal findings in the evaluation of sanity and competency. Tests that address broad personality issues such as judgment, ego strengths, impulse control, parenting ability, and object relations are sometimes administered. Questions of disposition after hospitalization can be clarified with a battery of personality tests that assess the patient's ability to tolerate stress, live independently, comply with therapy and benefit from outpatient treatment.

D. Common diagnostic issues that may be resolved by psychological testing include: identifying covert psychotic processes, distinguishing between functional psychoses and personality disorders, quantifying the degree of psychogenic overlay to a physical symptom, and distinguishing between depression and dementia. An initial battery of projective, empirical, and objective tests may reveal previously unsuspected organic brain disease requiring further investigation with neuropsychological testing (NPT) and neurologic evaluation. NPT should be included in the initial battery if organic disease is suggested by the clinical examination.

E. A broad battery of tests can be useful in determining specific strengths and weaknesses, suitability for supportive, insight-oriented, or behavioral psychotherapy, need for in- or outpatient treatment, and possible usefulness of medications in addition to psychological approaches.

F. NPT is the least intrusive means of characterizing organic brain disorders and the most objective means of quantifying the baseline in conditions that are likely to deteriorate, such as dementias. Practice effect (improved performance resulting from increasing familiarity with the test) can be controlled when tests are administered repeatedly. Baseline measures of psychosocial function selected from a comprehensive battery are useful in documenting the ongoing status of acute psychoses in order to determine whether the course is deteriorating, remitting, or static.

G. It is important to formulate questions as specifically as possible so that the psychologist may select the most appropriate test. The psychologist should be informed of the realistic range of possibilities so that he knows the limitations of his findings, can discuss test results in a way that is most likely to be helpful, and can decide whether a subspecialist (e.g., a neuropsychologist) is needed.

H. Written and verbal reports are usually provided rapidly to the referring professional. If the psychologist is present when test results are discussed with the patient or staff, unanticipated questions about the findings or their significance may be answered expeditiously.

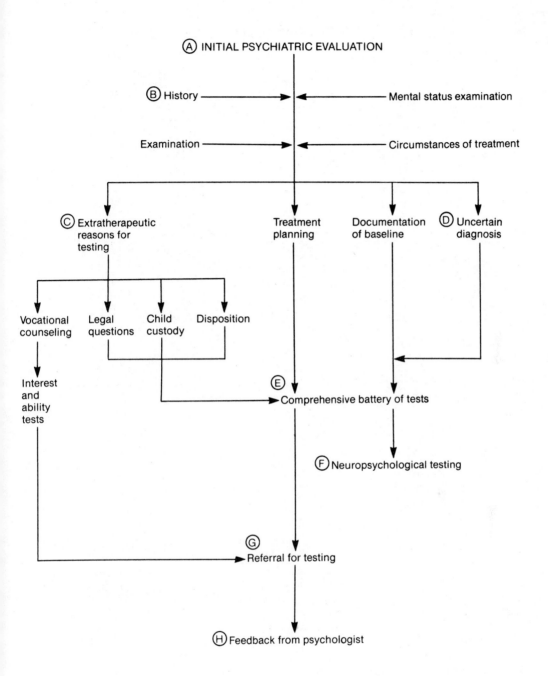

(A) INITIAL PSYCHIATRIC EVALUATION

(B) History ⟶ ⟵ Mental status examination

Examination ⟶ ⟵ Circumstances of treatment

(C) Extratherapeutic reasons for testing

Treatment planning

Documentation of baseline

(D) Uncertain diagnosis

Vocational counseling

Legal questions

Child custody

Disposition

Interest and ability tests

(E) Comprehensive battery of tests

(F) Neuropsychological testing

(G) Referral for testing

(H) Feedback from psychologist

TABLE 1   SOME ANTIPSYCHOTIC (NEUROLEPTIC) DRUGS

Drugs	Usual Daily Maintenance Dose	Sedative Properties	Anticholinergic Properties	EPS *
Phenothiazines				
Chlorpromazine (Thorazine)	75 – 400 mg	Strong	Strong	Low
Thioridazine (Mellaril)	75 – 400 mg	Moderate	Very strong	Low
Trifluoperazine (Stelazine)	4 – 20 mg	Low	Moderate	Moderate
Fluphenazine (Prolixin)	4 – 20 mg			
Butyrophenone				
Haloperidol (Haldol)	5 – 40 mg	Low	Low	High
Thioxanthenes				
Thiothixene (Navane)	20 – 30 mg	Low	Moderate	High
Dihydroindolones				
Molindone (Moban)	20 – 100 mg	Moderate	Strong	Moderate
Dibenzoxazepines				
Loxapine (Loxitane)	25 – 100 mg	Moderate	Low	High

* Extrapyramidal side effects

TABLE 2   SOME SIDE EFFECTS OF PSYCHIATRIC DRUGS

Syndrome	Causative Medications	Manifestations
CNS depression	Sedatives, tranquilizers, antihistamines, some neuroleptics and antidepressants	Lethargy, drowsiness, depression, decreased activity
Paradoxical reactions	Tranquilizers and sedatives	Agitation, restlessness, excitement, insomnia, psychosis
Anticholinergic symptoms	Antihistamines, some neuroleptics and antidepressants	Fever, tachycardia, blurred vision, dry mouth, constipation, urinary retention, psychosis
Alpha adrenergic blockade	Neuroleptics and antidepressants	Orthostatic hypotension; interference with alpha adrenergic drugs
Retinitis pigmentosa	Thioridazine	Pigmentary retinopathy with thioridazine >800 mg/day
Peripheral neuropathy	Tricyclic antidepressants, disulfiram, carbamazepine, or depression with psychomotor slowing	Motor, sensory, and reflex changes in lower extremities
Extrapyramidal syndromes Parkinsonism	Neuroleptics	Rigidity, tremor, mask–like face, hypersalivation, shuffling gate, appearing within month, abating within 6 months
Acute dystonia		Torticollis, oculogyric crisis, opisthotonus, dystonic movements
Akathesia		Inner restlessness, inability to sit still, leg movements, fidgeting, agitation
Tardive dyskinesia	Neuroleptics	Involuntary abnormal movements of face and tongue, choreoathetoid movements of limbs and trunk; signs often appear after a decrease in dosage.
Catatonia	Antipsychotics, amphetamines, aspirin, ACTH, porphyria, diabetic acidosis, hypercalcemia, hepatic encephalopathy, pellagra, glomerulonephritis	Waxy flexibility, negativism, withdrawal, parkinsonism mimicking catatonic psychosis.
Neuroleptic malignant syndrome	Haloperidol, thioridazine, sedative–hypnotics	Muscular rigidity, hyperthermia, stupor, coma, tachycardia, labile blood pressure, respiratory distress, diaphoresis, incontinence. Develops over 1–3 days, hours to months after starting haloperidol or thioridazine, or after withdrawal of sedative hypnotics. 20 – 30% fatality. Dantrolene is an effective treatment.
Irreversible mixed neurological syndrome	Lithium plus haloperidol or thioridazine	Fever, ataxia, lethargy, weakness, confusion, extrapyramidal syndromes, paralysis
Heat stroke	Anticholinergics, neuroleptics	Fever, decreased sweating, collapse. May occur in hot weather in patients taking anticholinergic drugs (decrease sweating) and neuroleptics (decrease thirst).
Skin and eye changes	Neuroleptics, especially chlorpromazine and thioridazine	Pigmentation of skin, lens, and cornea, lenticular opacities, with long–term and/or high–dose therapy

INDEX

in children, 170
in schizophrenia, 36
insomnia and, 90
memory loss and, 100
narcotics, 108
potential, in anxiety, 50
prescribing addictive drugs, 110
self-destructive behavior and, 48
withdrawal syndromes, 106, 112
See also specific drugs
Drug adulterants, 112
Drug taking
detoxification, 72, 73
emotional factor in, 70
side effects, 179
Drug-induced nightmares, 86
Dysthymic disorder, 46

Eating, binge, 134
Ejaculation
premature, 124
retarded, 126
Electroconvulsive therapy
for agitation, 14
for attempted suicide, 16
in atypical psychosis, 32
in depression, 58, 60
in incipient schizophrenia, 41
in mania, 28, 42
Electroencephalography
and atypical psychosis, 32
and bad dreams, 87
and delirium, 96, 100
and dementia, 98
and sleep disturbances, 89
Emergency treatment, in acute drug syndrome, 104
Emesis, for suicide by overdose, 20
Enuresis, 88
Epilepsy, 88
Epileptiform abnormalities, 32
Erectile dysfunction, 114
Exhibitionism, 128
Extrapyramidal syndromes, from neuroleptics, 179
Eye changes, from neuroleptics, 179

Factitious disorders, 34, 82, 84, 100
Family
in child abuse, 154
in couples therapy, 174
of alcoholic, 102
of child using drugs or alcohol, 170
of chronic schizophrenic, 36
of chronically ill patient, 80
of patient with dementia, 98
of pregnant patient, 78
of runaway child, 160
of socially withdrawn child, 168

of suicidal adolescent, 148
of suicidal child, 162
problems, and atypical physical symptoms, 70
Fear
anger and, 2
noncompliance and, 8
school phobia and, 164
treatment refusal and, 10
Febrile illness
and bad dreams, 86
and delirium, 96
Fees, payment failure, 6, 7
Female orgasmic dysfunction, 116
Fetishism, 128
Financial problems with patient, 6
Fluoxetine, 66, 67
Fluphenazine, 178
Flurazepam, 69, 94, 95
Fluvoxamine, 66, 67
Fugue, 100

Gains, secondary, 82
Gender identity, 166
Grief, 54, 56
and dying patient, 76
and unexplained somatic complaints, 84
in children, 156
See also Mourning

Hallucination
acute psychosis and, 30
memory loss and, 101
physical complaint and, 84
Hallucinogens
and acute drug and alcohol syndromes, 112, 113
and acute drug syndromes, 104
See also Drug abuse
Haloperidol, 65, 178
and agitation, 14, 15
and borderline personality, 140
and dementia, 98
with lithium, 44
contraindications, 28
Hearing impairment, in children, 168
Heat stroke, from anticholinergics or neuroleptics, 179
Homicide
risk of, 18
threat of, 18–19, 24
See also Aggression; Anger; Dangerous behavior
Homosexuality, 13, 120, 166
Hospitalization
"against medical advice" threat, 172
during pregnancy, 78
for acute psychosis, 30
for acute schizophrenia, 36

and depression, 58, 60, 64, 65
and sleepiness, 92
See also specific drugs
Morning sickness, 78
Motherhood, teenage, 166
Mourning, 54, 76
in children, 156
chronic illness and, 80
dementia and, 98
Multiple personality, 100
Munchausen's syndrome. *See* Factitious
disorders
Murderous impulses. *See* Homicide
Musculoskeletal dysfunction, and insomnia, 90

Naloxone, and acute drug syndromes, 105
Narcolepsy, 92
Narcotics, 112
abuse, 108. *See also* Drug abuse
and acute drug and alcohol syndromes,
112, 113
contaminants, 112
prescription of, 110
withdrawal, 106, 108
Nausea and vomiting, with pregnancy, 78
Neuroleptic drugs, 178
and acute drug syndromes, 104
and acute psychosis, 30
and agitation, 14
and anxiety, 172
and atypical psychoses, 32
and borderline personality, 140
and chronic schizophrenia, 36, 38
and depression, 59, 65
and incipient schizophrenic psychosis, 40
and mania, 42
and psychoses, 28, 29
in pregnancy, 74
side effects, 179
See also specific drugs and groups of drugs
Neuroleptic malignant syndrome, 179
Neuropsychological testing, 176
Newborn, narcotic withdrawal and, 108
Nightmares, 86
Nocturnal myoclonus, 90
Nocturnal seizures, 88
Nomifensine, 66, 67
Noncompliance. *See* Compliance/
noncompliance
Nortriptyline, 63

Obesity, 136
Oneiroid states, 32
Organic affective syndrome, 42
Organic brain syndromes
acute, 96
agitation with, 14
atypical physical symptoms and, 70
chronically ill and, 80, 81

depression and, 56
deviant sexual behavior and, 129
diagnosis of, 30, 32, 34, 42
drug taking and, 70, 100
self-destructive behavior with, 48
somatic complaints and, 84
threats to leave hospital prematurely, 172
See also Delirium
Orgasm, in women, 116
Overdose, drugs, and suicide attempt, 21. *See
also* Drug abuse
Over-the-counter drugs, 112
Oxazepam, 50, 69

Pain
benign intractable, 72
in dying patient, 76
Panic, 50, 52
and dying patient, 76
Paradoxical reactions to drugs, 179
Paraldehyde, and agitation, 15
Paranoid psychosis, 29, 32
and acute drug syndromes, 104
and bizarre or unusual thinking, 34
Paraphilias, 128
Paraphrenia, late-onset, 32
Parenting, bonding in, 152
Parkinsonism, from neuroleptics, 179
PCP intoxication, 104
Pedophilia, 128
Penile Doppler studies, and sexual dysfunction,
118
Pentobarbital, 106
Peripheral neuropathy syndrome, 179
Personality change, 34
Personality disorder
and agitation, 15
and bizarre or unusual thinking, 34
and depression, 46, 56
and self-destructive behavior, 48
and substance abuse in childhood, 170
antisocial, 138
borderline, 140
Phenelzine, 65, 134
Phenobarbital, 106
Phenothiazines, 178
Phentolamine, and acute drug syndromes, 104
Phobias, 50, 52
following rape, 23
Physical symptoms
atypical, 70
psychiatric evaluation, 70
Physician
and threatening patient, 18, 24
anger with, 2–3
payment delinquency and, 6–7
reaction to homosexual patient, 12
Physician-patient relationship
and borderline personality, 140

and chronic psychosis, 38
and disturbed behavior during pregnancy, 74
and dying patient, 76
and homosexuality, 120
compliance/noncompliance and, 8
treatment refusal and, 10, 172
Physostigmine, and acute drug syndromes, 105
Pimozide, 32
Poisoning, emergency management, 20
Pregnancy
    alcohol intake in, 74
    disturbed behavior during, 74
    hyperemesis gravidarum in, 78
    psychotropic drugs during, 74
    self-destructive behavior with, 74
Premorbid functioning, 28
Primary gain, 82
Promiscuity, in adolescence, 166
Propranolol, 15, 28, 50, 68, 69, 98
Protriptyline
    and depression, 58, 63
    and sleepiness, 92, 93
Psychoactive substances, insanity plea and, 146
Psychogenic amnesia, 100
Psychogenic illness, 84
Psychogenic pain disorder, 46, 70
Psychological testing, 176
Psychoses
    atypical, 32
    characteristics of, 28, 29
    See also headings under specific disorders and Psychosis
Psychosis
    acute, 30
    and antisocial personality, 138
    and atypical physical symptoms, 70
    and bizarre or unusual thinking, 34
    and borderline personality, 140
    and child runaways, 160
    and depression, 61
    and memory loss, 100
    and unexplained somatic complaints, 84
    atypical, 32
    chronic, 38
    cycloid, 32
    in medical illness, 38
    incipient schizophrenic, 40
    paranoid. *See* Paranoid disorder
    with pregnancy, 74
Psychosocial crisis, 34
Psychosomatic syndromes, 70
Psychotherapy outpatient, 19
Pyrodoxine, and depression, 65

Rape victim, 23
    homosexual, 120
Reality, loss of, 30
Reality testing, 31

Restless leg syndrome, 90
Reactive psychosis, brief, 28, 30, 32
Restraint
    for acute psychosis, 30
    for agitation, 14
    for mania, 42
    for threatening patient, 24
Retardation, 168
Retinitis pigmentosa syndrome, 179
Running away from home, 160

Sadism, 128
Schizoaffective disorder, 28, 29, 32
Schizophrenia
    agitation and, 14
    atypical psychoses and, 32
    bizarre thinking and, 34
    characteristics, 28, 29
    chronic, 36
    depression and, 46, 56
    in children, 162
    incidence, 36
    incipient, 40
    medical problems in, 36
    memory loss and, 100
    psychotic behavior breakthroughs, 36
    rehabilitation in, 40
    relapse rate, 36
Schizophreniform disorders, 29, 32
Schizotypal personality, 34
School, behavior problems in, 158
School phobia, 158, 164
Secondary gain, 82, 84
Seductive behavior, 12
Self-destructive behavior
    anorexia nervosa, 132
    chronic severe, 48
    involuntary hospitalization, 142
    with pregnancy, 74
    See also Suicide
Self-mutilation, 48
Separation anxiety
    childhood depression and, 156
    in hospitalized child, 168
    school behavior problems and, 158
    school phobia and, 164
Sex change, 166
Sexual behavior
    after rape, 22
    deviant, 128
    disinterest in, 122
    dysfunction and, 118
    female orgasm and, 116
    homosexuality, 120
    impotence and, 114
    in adolescence, 166
    premature ejaculation, 124
    retarded ejaculation, 126
    seductive, 12

vaginismus and, 130
Simulation of illness. *See* Factitious disorders
Sexual dysfunction, approach to, 118
Skin changes, from neuroleptics, 179
Sleep
    apnea, 90, 92
    attacks, 92
    paralysis, 92
    sleep-related dysfunctions, 88
    terrors, 86
    See also Insomnia
Sleep laboratory evaluation, 91, 93
Sleepiness, excessive daytime, 92
Sleeping pills
    and insomnia, 90
    prescribing, 110
Sleepwalking, 86, 88
Social withdrawal, 168
Sociopathic behavior, 34
Somatic complaints, unexplained, 84
Somatic therapies, and acute psychosis, 31
Somatoform disorders, 46, 70
Speech, bizarre or grandiose, and memory loss, 101
Splitting, and borderline personality, 140
Spouse abuse, 26–27
Stage fright, and anxiety, 50
Stimulants
    and alcohol syndromes, 112, 113
    and behavior problems in school, 158
    and depression, 65
    and sleepiness, 93
    central nervous system, and acute drug withdrawal, 106
Stress
    antisocial personality and, 139
    anxiety with, 52
    borderline personality and, 140
    chronic pain with, 72
    chronic psychosis and, 38
    conversion symptoms and, 82
    incipient schizophrenia and, 40
    insomnia and, 90
    mania and, 42
    memory loss and, 100
    nightmares and, 86
    seductive behavior and, 12
    sleep-related dysfunctions and, 88
    unexplained somatic complaints and, 84, 85
Stress disorder, post-traumatic, 50, 52
Stupor, and acute drug syndromes, 105
Substance abuse. *See* Alcohol abuse; Drug abuse
Suicide
    acute attempt, 16
    and anorexia nervosa, 133
    as self-destructive behavior, 48
    childhood risk, 162
    depression and, 56, 58
    drug abstinence syndromes and, 106
    grief and, 54
    in adolescent, 148
    overdose emergency management, 20
    risk of, 16
    with pregnancy, 74
    See also Anger; Self-destructive behavior

T_3. *See* Triiodothyronine
Tachycardia
    and acute drug syndromes, 105
    and anxiety, 50
    as self-destructive behavior, 48
Tardive dyskinesia
    from neuroleptics, 179
Teeth grinding, during sleep, 88
Temazepam, 69, 94, 95
Terminal illness, 76
Testing, psychological, 176
Testosterone level, and sexual dysfunction, 119
Thiothixine, 178
Thioridazine, 64, 65
    as cause of retinitis pigmentosa syndrome, 179
    contraindications with lithium, 28
Thioxanthenes, 178
Thought disorders, 30, 34
Thyroxine, 32
Tongue biting, during sleep, 88
Tranquilizers
    contraindication in acute drug syndromes, 105
    for agitation, 14
    in alcoholism, 102
    prescribing, 110
Transference, anger and, 2
Transsexualism, 166
Transvestism, 128, 166
Tranylcypromine, 65, 134
Trazodone, 58, 62, 63
Treatment
    failure to respond to, 9
    refusal of, 10, 11
    Tremor, and anxiety, 50
    Triazolam, 69, 94, 95
Tricyclic antidepressants, 50, 52, 59
    and bulimia, 134
    and nightmares, 86
    nonresponse to, 60
Trifluoperazine, 178
Triiodothyronine, and antidepressants, 64, 65
Trimipramine, 63
L-Tryptophan, and depression, 65
Tyramine, contraindication with MAO inhibitors, 58, 134

Vaginal smear test, and sexual dysfunction, 119